Emerging Trends in Clinical Pharmacy:

Exploring the Evolving Landscape

www.lulu.com
Lulu Press, Inc
627 Davis Drive, Suite 300,
Morrisville, NC 27560.

Author Affiliations

Dr. Hemraj Singh Rajput,
Associate Professor,
Department of Pharmacy Practice,
Sumandeep Vidyapeeth Deemed to be University,
Waghodia, Vadodara, Gujarat, India.

Dr. Rajesh Hadia,
Assistant Professor,
Department of Pharmacy Practice,
Sumandeep Vidyapeeth Deemed to be University,
Waghodia, Vadodara, Gujarat, India.

Dr. Varunsingh Saggu,
Assistant Professor,
Department of Pharmacy Practice,
Sumandeep Vidyapeeth Deemed to be University,
Waghodia, Vadodara, Gujarat, India.

Dr. Cyril Sajan,
Assistant Professor,
Department of Pharmacy Practice,
Sumandeep Vidyapeeth Deemed to be University,
Waghodia, Vadodara, Gujarat, India.

First Printing: 2023
ISBN: 978-1-312-26662-9
Copyright License @ Dr. Hemraj Singh Rajput

This book has been published with all reasonable efforts to make the material error-free after the author's consent. No part of this book shall be used or reproduced in any manner, without the author's permission, except for brief quotations embodied in critical articles and reviews.

The Author of this book is solely responsible and liable for its content, including but not limited to the views, representations, descriptions, statements, information, opinions, and references ["Content"]. The Content of this book shall not constitute or be construed or deemed to reflect the opinion or expression of the Publisher or Editor. Neither the Publisher nor Editor endorse or approve the Content of this book or guarantee the reliability, accuracy, or completeness of the Content published herein and do not make any representations or warranties of any kind, express or implied, including but not limited to the implied warranties of merchantability, fitness for a particular purpose. The Publisher and Editor shall not be liable whatsoever for any errors or omissions, whether such errors or omissions result from negligence, accident, or any other cause or claims for loss or damages of any kind, including without limitation, indirect or consequential loss or damage arising out of use, inability to use, or about the reliability, accuracy or sufficiency of the information contained in this book. This book was written based on Intelligence with the support of various sources.

Emerging Trends in Clinical Pharmacy: Exploring the Evolving Landscape

By

Dr. Hemraj Singh Rajput,

Dr. Rajesh Hadia,

Dr. Varunsingh Saggu,

Dr. Cyril Sajan.

2023

About the Authors

Dr. Hemraj Singh Rajput, *B. Pharm & Pharm. D* is an Associate Professor with 7 years of experience in the Pharmacy Practice Department. He authored 30 paper publications, including research, review, and case reports in national and international journals. He also presented and participated in various conferences, workshops, seminars, webinars, symposiums, etc. He is a member of APTI. He gave a reputable talk at GSPC. He also organized 3 national-level conferences. His focus research area is clinical pharmacy, drug-drug interactions, and public health.

Dr. Rajesh Hadia, *Pharm. D*, an Assistant Professor, authored 40 paper publications, including research, review, and case reports in national and international journals, and wrote 15 book chapters. He also presented and participated in various national and international conferences, workshops, seminars, webinars, symposiums, etc. He has been awarded the best paper at APTICON-2022. He is a member of APTI and a reviewer for esteemed journals. He has excellence in clinical pharmacy services and a commitment to promoting rational medication use and upholding ethical research practices.

Dr. Varunsingh Saggu, *Pharm. D,* an Assistant Professor with 3 years of teaching experience and 2 years as a clinical pharmacologist at the Hospital. He authored 5 research, review, and case report paper publications in national and international journals. He is an expert at giving hands-on training on drug-based decisions. His research expertise includes pharmacovigilance, clinical research, therapeutic drug monitoring, and antibiotic stewardship.

Dr. Cyril Sajan, *Pharm. D,* an Assistant Professor with 2 years of teaching experience and 1 year in the pharmaceutical industry. He authored 20 paper publications, including research, review, and case study papers in national and international journals, and wrote 10 book chapters. His research interests include pharmacovigilance, clinical research, therapeutic drug monitoring, and Toxicology.

About Book

Emerging Trends in Clinical Pharmacy: Exploring the Evolving Landscape" is a comprehensive book by leading experts, covering cutting-edge research, precision medicine, AI applications, and patient-centered care. It offers multidisciplinary insights, real-world case studies, and ethical considerations for pharmacy professionals and researchers. The book is a vital resource for staying up-to-date with the ever-changing field of clinical pharmacy and predicting future directions in healthcare.

Emerging Trends in Clinical Pharmacy: Exploring the Evolving Landscape

Table of Contents

1. Introduction 1
    1.1 Background 3
    1.2 Objectives 5
    1.3 Scope of the Study 7
    1.4 Methodology 9
2. Overview of Clinical Pharmacy 11
    2.1 Definition and Evolution of Clinical Pharmacy 11
    2.2 Role of Clinical Pharmacists 13
    2.3 Importance in Healthcare 15
3. Traditional Clinical Pharmacy Practices 18
    3.1 Medication Therapy Management 18
    3.2 Pharmaceutical Care 21
    3.3 Drug Information Services 24
    3.4 Clinical Decision Support Systems 26
    3.5 Medication Reconciliation 28
4. Technological Advances in Clinical Pharmacy 31
    4.1 Electronic Health Records 31
    4.2 Telepharmacy 33
    4.3 Clinical Pharmacy Software 36
    4.4 Pharmacy Automation Systems 38
    4.5 Mobile Applications in Clinical Pharmacy 40
5. Precision Medicine and Personalized Pharmacotherapy 43
    5.1 Genomics and Pharmacogenomics 43
    5.2 Biomarkers in Clinical Decision Making 45

5.3 Individualized Treatment Approaches 47

5.4 Challenges and Opportunities 50

6. Integration of Pharmacists in Interprofessional Healthcare Teams 53

6.1 Collaborative Practice Models 53

6.2 Team-Based Care and Communication 55

6.3 Improved Patient Outcomes 57

6.4 Barriers and Facilitators 60

7. Emerging Roles for Clinical Pharmacists 63

7.1 Pharmacogeneticists 63

7.2 Pharmacovigilance Specialists 65

7.3 Clinical Pharmacy Consultants 67

7.3 Clinical Pharmacy Consultants 69

7.4 Transitions of Care Pharmacists 71

7.5 Clinical Research Pharmacists 73

8. Contemporary Issues in Clinical Pharmacy 77

8.1 Medication Safety and Quality Assurance 77

8.3 Pharmaceutical Industry Influence 81

8.4 Medication Adherence Challenges 84

8.5 Global Health and Access to Medicines 86

9. Future Perspectives in Clinical Pharmacy 89

9.1 Artificial Intelligence and Machine Learning 89

9.2 Virtual Reality and Augmented Reality 91

9.3 Nanotechnology in Drug Delivery 93

9.4 Blockchain Technology in Pharmacy 95

9.5 Emerging Therapeutic Approaches 97

10. Clinical Pharmacy in Specialized Areas 100

- 10.1 Oncology Pharmacy 100
- 10.2 Critical Care Pharmacy 102
- 10.3 Pediatric Pharmacy 104
- 10.4 Geriatric Pharmacy 106
- 10.5 Ambulatory Care Pharmacy 108

11. Challenges and Opportunities for Clinical Pharmacists 111
- 11.1 Regulatory and Legal Considerations 111
- 11.2 Education and Training 113
- 11.3 Advancement and Recognition 116
- 11.4 Collaboration and Communication 118
- 11.5 Advocacy and Leadership 121

12. Conclusion 125
- 12.1 Summary of Key Findings 125
- 12.2 Implications for Clinical Pharmacy Practice 127
- 12.3 Recommendations for Future Research 129

References 132

Appendix 133
- Appendix A: Glossary of Terms 133
- Appendix B: Examples of Clinical Pharmacy Practice Models 137
- Appendix C: Survey Questionnaire for Clinical Pharmacists 140

Emerging Trends in Clinical Pharmacy: Exploring the Evolving Landscape

1. Introduction

Dr. Hemraj Singh Rajput

Clinical pharmacy is a field that continues to evolve and adapt to meet the changing needs of healthcare. Here are some emerging trends in clinical pharmacy that are shaping the evolving landscape:

Pharmacogenomics: Pharmacogenomics is the study of how an individual's genetic makeup influences their response to medications. It involves using genetic testing to determine the most effective and safe medications for patients based on their genetic profile. Clinical pharmacists are increasingly using pharmacogenomic information to personalize medication regimens and optimize treatment outcomes.

Medication Therapy Management (MTM): MTM is a patient-centered service provided by clinical pharmacists to optimize medication use and improve patient outcomes. It involves comprehensive medication reviews, identifying drug therapy problems, and developing individualized care plans. As healthcare systems focus more on patient-centered care and medication safety, the demand for MTM services is growing, and clinical pharmacists are playing a crucial role in providing these services.

Telepharmacy and Telehealth: The use of telepharmacy and telehealth technologies has expanded significantly in recent years. Clinical pharmacists can remotely provide medication-related services, including medication counseling, medication reviews, and monitoring patients' medication adherence. Telepharmacy and telehealth improve access to clinical pharmacy services, especially in rural or underserved areas, and enable pharmacists to reach a larger patient population.

Collaborative Practice: Collaborative practice models involve clinical pharmacists working closely with other healthcare providers, such as physicians, nurses, and advanced practice providers, to deliver comprehensive patient care. This team-based approach enhances medication management, promotes medication safety, and improves patient outcomes. Clinical pharmacists are increasingly being integrated into various healthcare settings, including primary care clinics, hospitals, and specialty clinics.

Specialty Pharmacy: Specialty medications, used to treat complex and chronic conditions, have become more prevalent in recent years. Clinical pharmacists specializing in this field provide specialized services, including medication management, patient education, and coordination of care. They work closely with patients, healthcare providers, and payers to ensure safe and effective use of specialty medications and optimize patient outcomes.

Data Analytics and Evidence-Based Practice: The availability of vast amounts of healthcare data has opened up new opportunities for clinical pharmacists to utilize data analytics and evidence-based practice. By analyzing patient data, clinical pharmacists can identify patterns, optimize medication therapies, and contribute to population health management efforts. They also play a critical role in translating research evidence into practice and implementing best practices for medication use.

Continuous Professional Development: Clinical pharmacy is a dynamic field with advancements in drug therapies and healthcare delivery. To keep up with these changes, clinical pharmacists are engaging in continuous professional development activities, such as attending conferences, participating in webinars, and pursuing advanced certifications. This ongoing learning ensures that clinical pharmacists remain current with the latest developments and provide the highest quality of care to patients.

Overall, the evolving landscape of clinical pharmacy is characterized by a shift towards personalized and patient-centered care, increased integration within healthcare teams, and the utilization of advanced technologies and data analytics. These trends highlight the expanding role of clinical pharmacists in improving medication outcomes and optimizing patient care.

1.1 Background

Clinical pharmacy is a specialized field of pharmacy practice that focuses on providing direct patient care, optimizing medication therapy, and ensuring safe and effective medication use. Clinical pharmacists work collaboratively with other healthcare professionals to manage medication-related issues, promote rational drug use, and improve patient outcomes.

The concept of clinical pharmacy emerged in the 1960s as a response to the increasing complexity of medication regimens and the need for pharmacists to have a more active role in patient care. Traditional pharmacy practice primarily involved dispensing medications, but clinical pharmacy expanded the role of pharmacists to encompass direct patient care activities.

Clinical pharmacists are trained to assess patients' medication needs, monitor drug therapy, identify and resolve medication-related problems, provide medication counseling, and educate patients about their medications. They work in various healthcare settings, including hospitals, clinics, ambulatory care centers, and community pharmacies.

Over the years, clinical pharmacy has evolved in response to advancements in medical knowledge, changes in healthcare delivery models, and the recognition of pharmacists as essential members of the healthcare team. The field has expanded beyond the hospital setting to encompass primary care, specialty care, and even remote or telepharmacy services.

Emerging Trends in Clinical Pharmacy: Exploring the Evolving Landscape

Clinical pharmacists now play integral roles in interdisciplinary healthcare teams, working alongside physicians, nurses, and other healthcare professionals. They contribute to medication selection, dosage optimization, monitoring for drug interactions or adverse effects, and providing evidence-based recommendations for medication therapy.

Furthermore, with the increasing prevalence of chronic diseases, complex drug regimens, and the advent of precision medicine, clinical pharmacists are utilizing pharmacogenomic testing and personalized medicine approaches to tailor medication therapies based on patient' genetic profiles.

The evolving landscape of clinical pharmacy is also influenced by advancements in technology, such as electronic health records (EHRs), telehealth platforms, and data analytics tools. These technologies facilitate communication, information sharing, and medication management across different healthcare settings, improving patient access to clinical pharmacy services and enhancing medication safety.

As healthcare systems strive to achieve better patient outcomes, reduce healthcare costs, and improve population health, the role of clinical pharmacy continues to expand and adapt. Clinical pharmacists are actively engaged in research, quality improvement initiatives, and professional development to stay abreast of emerging trends and best practices in medication therapy management.

In summary, clinical pharmacy is a dynamic and evolving field that focuses on optimizing medication therapy and improving patient outcomes. With its patient-centered approach, integration within healthcare teams and utilization of advanced technologies, clinical pharmacy plays a vital role in delivering safe, effective, and personalized medication care to patients.

1.2 Objectives

The objectives of clinical pharmacy can be summarized as follows:

Optimize Medication Therapy: Clinical pharmacists aim to ensure that patients receive the most appropriate medications for their conditions. This includes selecting the right drug, determining the optimal dosage, considering individual patient factors, and managing potential drug interactions or adverse effects. The objective is to achieve the best possible therapeutic outcomes while minimizing the risks associated with medication use.

Improve Patient Safety: Clinical pharmacists play a critical role in medication safety by identifying and preventing medication errors, adverse drug events, and drug interactions. They collaborate with healthcare teams to develop strategies for safe medication practices, promote medication reconciliation, and provide education to patients and healthcare professionals regarding medication safety measures.

Enhance Medication Adherence: Non-adherence to medication regimens is a common issue that can negatively impact treatment outcomes. Clinical pharmacists work with patients to address barriers to adherence and provide education on the importance of taking medications as prescribed. They may develop personalized adherence plans, offer reminder systems, and conduct medication counseling to support patients in maintaining proper medication adherence.

Provide Medication Education and Counseling: Clinical pharmacists are experts in medications and their proper use. They play a crucial role in educating patients about their medications, including dosage instructions, potential side effects, and precautions. They ensure that patients have a clear understanding of their treatment plan and empower them to make informed decisions about their medication therapy.

Collaborate with Healthcare Teams: Clinical pharmacists actively collaborate with other healthcare professionals, such as physicians, nurses, and allied health providers, to optimize patient care. They participate in interdisciplinary rounds, contribute to treatment planning, provide drug information and recommendations, and engage in shared decision-making processes. The objective is to ensure comprehensive and coordinated patient care.

Conduct Medication Reviews and Assessments: Clinical pharmacists perform medication reviews and assessments to identify potential drug therapy problems, such as inappropriate drug selection, suboptimal dosing, or medication-related adverse events. By evaluating medication regimens and patient-specific factors, they make recommendations to optimize drug therapy, improve efficacy, and minimize risks.

Engage in Research and Evidence-Based Practice: Clinical pharmacists contribute to the advancement of knowledge in the field through research activities. They participate in clinical trials, conduct medication-related research, and critically evaluate the available evidence to inform their practice. By staying updated with the latest research findings, clinical pharmacists ensure that their recommendations are based on the best available evidence.

Promote Quality Improvement: Clinical pharmacists actively engage in quality improvement initiatives to enhance medication-related processes and patient outcomes. They contribute to medication safety programs, participate in medication use evaluations, develop protocols and guidelines, and implement strategies to optimize medication management practices. The objective is to continually improve the quality and efficiency of medication use within healthcare settings.

Overall, the objectives of clinical pharmacy revolve around optimizing medication therapy, promoting patient safety, improving medication adherence, educating patients, collaborating with healthcare teams, conducting medication assessments, staying updated with evidence-based practices, and contributing to quality improvement efforts. These objectives collectively aim to deliver optimal patient care and improve health outcomes through effective medication management.

1.3 Scope of the Study

The scope of the study on emerging trends in clinical pharmacy and the evolving landscape can encompass various aspects within the field. Here are some areas that can be considered:

Emerging Practices and Services: The study can explore new and evolving practices and services offered by clinical pharmacists. This may include medication therapy management (MTM), pharmacogenomics, telepharmacy, collaborative practice models, specialty pharmacy, and other innovative approaches to patient care.

Integration in Healthcare Settings: The study examined the integration of clinical pharmacists within different healthcare settings, such as hospitals, clinics, primary care practices, specialty clinics, and ambulatory care centers. It can investigate the roles and responsibilities of clinical pharmacists in these settings and how they contribute to patient care.

Technology and Data Analytics: The study can focus on the use of technology, electronic health records (EHRs), telehealth platforms, and data analytics tools in clinical pharmacy practice. It can explore how these technologies are utilized to enhance medication management, improve communication and collaboration among healthcare providers, and optimize patient outcomes.

Patient-Centered Care: The study examine the patient-centered approach in clinical pharmacy and how it is implemented. It can explore patient education and counseling, medication adherence strategies, shared decision-making, and the impact of clinical pharmacists on patient satisfaction and health-related quality of life.

Collaborative Practice: The study can investigate the collaborative practice models in which clinical pharmacists work alongside other healthcare professionals. It can explore the nature of collaboration, interdisciplinary team dynamics, and the outcomes achieved through collaborative approaches to patient care.

Professional Development and Training: The study can explore the professional development and training opportunities available to clinical pharmacists. It can investigate continuing education, certification programs, advanced training in specialized areas, and the importance of staying updated with emerging trends and evidence-based practices.

Research and Evidence-Based Practice: The study examined the role of clinical pharmacists in research activities and evidence-based practice. It can explore their involvement in research studies, contribution to the literature, and the translation of research findings into clinical practice to improve patient outcomes.

Policy and Regulatory Considerations: The study can address policy and regulatory factors that impact the practice of clinical pharmacy. This may include scope of practice regulations, reimbursement models, legal and ethical considerations, and the influence of policy changes on the evolving landscape of clinical pharmacy.

It's important to note that the specific scope of the study can be further refined and tailored based on the research objectives, available resources, and the specific interests of the researcher or organization conducting the study.

1.4 Methodology

The methodology for studying emerging trends in clinical pharmacy and exploring the evolving landscape can involve various approaches and techniques. Here are some standard methods that can be utilized:

Literature Review: Conducting a comprehensive literature review is essential to gather information and gain an understanding of the existing research, studies, and publications related to the subject. This involves searching academic databases, scientific journals, conference proceedings, and other relevant sources to identify key trends, concepts, and findings in clinical pharmacy.

Surveys and Questionnaires: Designing and administering surveys or questionnaires to clinical pharmacists, healthcare professionals, and stakeholders can provide valuable insights into current practices, challenges, and emerging trends. This quantitative data collection method allows for the collection of a large sample size and facilitates statistical analysis.

Interviews and Focus Groups: Conducting interviews or focus groups with clinical pharmacists, healthcare professionals, and experts in the field can provide in-depth qualitative data. This method allows for open-ended discussions, exploration of individual experiences and perspectives, and the generation of rich insights into the evolving landscape of clinical pharmacy.

Case Studies: Examining real-world case studies and success stories can provide practical examples of how emerging trends in clinical pharmacy have been implemented and their impact on patient care. Case studies can involve analyzing specific programs, initiatives, or healthcare institutions that have adopted innovative practices in clinical pharmacy.

Data Analysis: Analyzing available data, such as electronic health records, patient outcomes data, or medication utilization data, can provide quantitative insights into the impact of emerging trends in clinical pharmacy. Data analysis techniques may include statistical analysis, data mining, and interpretation of patterns and trends.

Expert Panels and Delphi Technique: Engaging expert panels or using the Delphi technique can involve gathering a group of clinical pharmacy experts to provide their opinions and insights on emerging trends and the future direction of the field. This method allows for consensus building, identification of key areas of focus, and generation of expert recommendations.

Observation and Ethnographic Research: Conducting observations and ethnographic research in clinical pharmacy settings can provide a deep understanding of the daily practices, interactions, and challenges faced by clinical pharmacists. This method involves immersing oneself in the field, observing workflows, and documenting the experiences of healthcare professionals and patients.

Document Analysis: Analyzing relevant documents, guidelines, policies, and reports related to clinical pharmacy can provide insights into the regulatory landscape, professional standards, and the influence of policy changes on the field. This method involves reviewing official documents and extracting key information and themes.

It's important to select the most appropriate methodology or combination of methodologies based on the research objectives, available resources, and the nature of the research study. Additionally, ethical considerations should be considered, and necessary permissions and approvals should be obtained before conducting any research involving human subjects.

2. Overview of Clinical Pharmacy

Dr. Hemraj Singh Rajput

2.1 Definition and Evolution of Clinical Pharmacy

Clinical pharmacy can be defined as a specialized area of pharmacy practice that focuses on direct patient care, optimizing medication therapy, and ensuring safe and effective use of medications. Clinical pharmacists utilize their pharmaceutical knowledge, clinical skills, and patient-centered approach to provide individualized medication management and contribute to improved patient outcomes.

The concept of clinical pharmacy emerged in the 1960s as a response to the increasing complexity of medication regimens and the need for pharmacists to have a more active role in patient care. Prior to this, pharmacy practice primarily focused on dispensing medications without direct involvement in patient care.

The evolution of clinical pharmacy can be attributed to several factors:

- ✓ Advancements in Medications and Treatment: The development of new medications and treatment modalities led to increased complexity in drug therapy. Clinical pharmacists recognized the need to have a comprehensive understanding of medications and their impact on patient health, which propelled the evolution of clinical pharmacy.
- ✓ Shifting Healthcare Paradigm: The healthcare industry witnessed a shift towards patient-centered care, emphasizing the importance of individualized treatment plans and improved outcomes. Clinical pharmacy emerged as a field that focused on tailoring medication therapy to meet the specific needs of patients and optimizing their health outcomes.

- ✓ Pharmacist Professionalism and Expanding Roles: Pharmacists started to assert their expertise and professional autonomy, recognizing the need to expand their roles beyond medication dispensing. Clinical pharmacy provided pharmacists with an opportunity to use their pharmaceutical knowledge and clinical skills to directly impact patient care.
- ✓ Collaborative Healthcare Approach: The importance of interprofessional collaboration in healthcare became increasingly recognized. Clinical pharmacy integrated pharmacists into healthcare teams, facilitating collaboration with other healthcare professionals to optimize patient care and medication therapy.

Over the years, clinical pharmacy has continued to evolve in response to advancements in medical knowledge, changes in healthcare delivery models, and the recognition of pharmacists as essential members of the healthcare team. The field has expanded beyond the hospital setting to encompass primary care, specialty care, and community-based practices.

Clinical pharmacists now engage in activities such as medication therapy management (MTM), medication reconciliation, pharmacogenomics, telepharmacy, and collaborative practice models. They actively contribute to patient care by conducting medication reviews, providing medication counseling, monitoring therapy, and participating in shared decision-making with patients and other healthcare professionals.

Furthermore, clinical pharmacists are involved in research, quality improvement initiatives, and evidence-based practice to enhance medication management and patient outcomes continually. Through continuous professional development and training, they stay updated with the latest advancements, guidelines, and therapeutic approaches.

Overall, the definition and evolution of clinical pharmacy reflect the field's adaptation to meet the changing healthcare landscape, emphasizing patient-centered care, interprofessional collaboration, and the optimization of medication therapy to improve patient outcomes.

2.2 Role of Clinical Pharmacists

The role of clinical pharmacists is multifaceted and encompasses various responsibilities within the healthcare system. Here are some key roles and functions performed by clinical pharmacists:

Medication Therapy Management: Clinical pharmacists are involved in comprehensive medication therapy management. They assess patients' medication needs, review medication regimens, identify drug therapy problems, and recommend optimizing therapy. This includes medication selection, dosage adjustment, monitoring for adverse effects, and addressing medication adherence issues.

Collaborative Patient Care: Clinical pharmacists work collaboratively with other healthcare professionals, including physicians, nurses, and allied health providers, as part of the healthcare team. They actively participate in interdisciplinary rounds, contribute to treatment planning, and provide medication-related expertise to ensure comprehensive patient care.

Medication Counseling and Education: Clinical pharmacists play a vital role in patient education and counseling. They inform patients about their medications, including proper usage, potential side effects, and precautions. They address patients' concerns, provide guidance on medication adherence, and empower patients to participate in their healthcare actively.

Medication Safety and Adverse Event Monitoring: Clinical pharmacists are responsible for monitoring medication safety and identifying and preventing adverse drug events (ADEs). They conduct medication reconciliation, review medication orders for appropriateness, monitor for interactions, and contribute to strategies for preventing medication errors.

Pharmacotherapy Consultation: Clinical pharmacists provide pharmacotherapy consultation services to healthcare professionals. They assist in selecting appropriate medications, determining optimal dosages, and developing evidence-based treatment plans. Their expertise in drug interactions, pharmacokinetics, and therapeutic guidelines helps inform decision-making for complex patient cases.

Pharmacovigilance and Drug Information: Clinical pharmacists actively monitor and report adverse drug reactions and events. They contribute to pharmacovigilance activities by identifying, documenting, and reporting ADEs to regulatory bodies. Additionally, they serve as drug information resources, providing accurate and up-to-date information on medications to healthcare professionals and patients.

Research and Evidence-Based Practice: Clinical pharmacists engage in research activities, clinical trials, and evidence-based practice to contribute to advancements in medication therapy and patient care. They critically evaluate research literature, apply findings to clinical practice, and participate in quality improvement initiatives to enhance medication management processes.

Specialty Pharmacy Services: Clinical pharmacists may specialize in various areas, such as cardiology, oncology, infectious diseases, or pediatrics. They provide specialized medication management services in these specialty areas, including disease-specific medication protocols, patient counseling, and monitoring for treatment-related complications.

Continuous Professional Development and Education: Clinical pharmacists are committed to lifelong learning and professional development. They stay updated with the latest advancements in pharmacotherapy, guidelines, and therapeutic approaches through continuing education, attending conferences, and pursuing advanced certifications.

The role of clinical pharmacists is dynamic and continues to evolve with advancements in healthcare and the increasing complexity of medication therapy. Their expertise in medications, patient care, and interprofessional collaboration positions them as essential healthcare team members, contributing to improved patient outcomes and medication safety.

2.3 Importance in Healthcare

Clinical pharmacists play a vital role in healthcare due to their unique expertise in medications and their impact on patient outcomes. Here are several reasons highlighting the importance of clinical pharmacists in healthcare:

Medication Optimization: Clinical pharmacists are essential in optimizing medication therapy. They have in-depth knowledge of medications, including their efficacy, safety profiles, and potential drug interactions. By assessing individual patient characteristics, clinical pharmacists can tailor medication regimens, select the most appropriate drugs, and optimize dosages to achieve optimal therapeutic outcomes.

Medication Safety and Adverse Event Prevention: Clinical pharmacists ensure medication safety and prevent adverse drug events (ADEs). They conduct medication reviews, monitor for potent drug interactions, identify medication errors, and provide recommendations to minimize risks. Their expertise helps prevent medication-related harm and enhances patient safety.

Medication Education and Counseling: Clinical pharmacists are excellent medication education and counseling resources. They inform patients about their medications, including proper usage, potential side effects, and precautions. By offering clear and concise explanations, clinical pharmacists empower patients to make informed decisions about their treatment and improve medication adherence.

Interprofessional Collaboration: Clinical pharmacists collaborate with other healthcare professionals to provide comprehensive patient care. They actively participate in interdisciplinary rounds, contribute to treatment planning, and provide medication-related expertise to ensure safe and effective medication use. Their input helps optimize medication therapy and improves patient outcomes.

Medication Adherence Support: Non-adherence to medication regimens significantly affects patient outcomes. Clinical pharmacists play a crucial role in promoting medication adherence. They assess barriers to compliance, educate patients on the importance of taking medications as prescribed, and provide strategies to enhance loyalty, such as reminder systems or simplified medication schedules.

Chronic Disease Management: With the increasing prevalence of chronic diseases, clinical pharmacists are crucial in managing complex medication regimens. They collaborate with healthcare teams to develop comprehensive treatment plans, provide ongoing monitoring, and adjust medications as needed. Clinical pharmacists contribute to the optimization of medication therapies for improved disease management.

Cost-Effective Medication Use: Clinical pharmacists know medication costs, formulary restrictions, and therapeutic alternatives. They help identify cost-effective treatment options without compromising efficacy or safety. Clinical pharmacists contribute to rational drug utilization and cost containment by considering the economic aspects of medication use.

Research and Evidence-Based Practice: Clinical pharmacists actively engage in research activities and evidence-based practice. They critically evaluate the available literature, contribute to clinical trials, and translate research findings into practice. This commitment to evidence-based medicine ensures that patient care is based on the best available evidence and fosters continuous improvement in healthcare.

Quality Improvement: Clinical pharmacists actively participate in quality improvement initiatives. They contribute to medication safety programs, implement protocols and guidelines, and develop strategies to enhance medication management processes. Their expertise helps identify areas for improvement and implement interventions to improve the quality of patient care.

Overall, the importance of clinical pharmacists in healthcare lies in their unique expertise in medications, patient care, and collaboration with other healthcare professionals. They optimize medication therapy, ensure medication safety, improve patient outcomes, and promote cost-effective medication use. By playing a critical role in various aspects of medication management, clinical pharmacists enhance the overall quality of care and patient safety in healthcare settings.

3. Traditional Clinical Pharmacy Practices

Dr. Hemraj Singh Rajput

3.1 Medication Therapy Management

Traditional clinical pharmacy practices encompass a broad range of activities that optimize medication therapy and ensure patient safety. Medication Therapy Management (MTM) is a critical component of traditional clinical pharmacy practices. Let's explore the relationship between traditional clinical pharmacy practices and MTM in more detail.

Traditional clinical pharmacy practices involve the following:

Medication Review and Assessment: Clinical pharmacists thoroughly review patients' medication regimens, assessing appropriateness, drug interactions, and potential adverse effects. They evaluate the medications in the context of the patient's medical history, allergies, and individual characteristics.

Medication Monitoring: Clinical pharmacists actively monitor patients' responses to medication therapy. They assess medication efficacy, evaluate for adverse effects or toxicities, and make appropriate adjustments to optimize treatment. Monitoring includes patient follow-ups, laboratory test interpretation, and medication adherence assessments.

Medication Education and Counseling: Clinical pharmacists educate and counsel patients regarding their medications. They explain proper usage, potential side effects, and precautions. Patient counseling promotes understanding, addresses concerns, and improves medication adherence.

Medication Safety and Adverse Event Prevention: Clinical pharmacists ensure medication safety and prevent adverse drug events

(ADEs). They conduct medication reconciliation, review prescriptions for accuracy, assess for potential errors, and monitor for medication-related adverse effects.

Collaborative Patient Care: Clinical pharmacists collaborate with healthcare teams to optimize patient care. They participate in interdisciplinary rounds, communicate medication-related recommendations, and contribute to treatment planning. Collaborative patient care ensures comprehensive and coordinated medication therapy.

Medication Therapy Management (MTM) is a patient-centered service clinical pharmacists provide to optimize medication use, improve medication adherence, and enhance patient outcomes. MTM involves a comprehensive approach to medication management that goes beyond the traditional dispensing of medications. Here are critical aspects of Medication Therapy Management:

Comprehensive Medication Review: Clinical pharmacists conduct a thorough review of a patient's complete medication regimen, including prescription medications, over-the-counter drugs, herbal supplements, and dietary supplements. They assess the appropriateness of the medications, evaluate the potential for drug interactions or duplications, and identify any drug-related problems.

Medication Optimization: Based on the comprehensive review, clinical pharmacists recommend optimizing medication therapy. This includes adjusting dosages, switching medications, discontinuing unnecessary medications, and selecting appropriate alternatives. The goal is to ensure that the patient is on the most effective and safest medication regimen.

Medication Adherence Assessment and Support: Clinical pharmacists evaluate a patient's medication adherence and identify barriers to observation, such as complex regimens, side effects, or cost-related issues. They provide patient education and counseling to promote understanding of the medications, address concerns, and develop strategies to enhance medication adherence. This may involve adherence aids, reminder systems, or personalized adherence plans.

Medication Safety Monitoring: Clinical pharmacists monitor for medication-related adverse effects, drug interactions, and potential risks. They collaborate with healthcare teams to identify and manage adverse drug reactions, evaluate laboratory values, and monitor the patient's medication response. This proactive monitoring helps ensure patient safety and minimize the occurrence of medication-related harm.

Patient Education and Counseling: Clinical pharmacists are crucial in educating patients about their medications. They provide information on medication purpose, proper administration, potential side effects, and precautions. Clinical pharmacists address patient questions and concerns and empower patients to actively participate in their medication management, improving medication knowledge and self-care skills.

Care Coordination and Collaboration: Clinical pharmacists collaborate with other healthcare professionals, such as physicians, nurses, and caregivers, to provide coordinated and patient-centered care. They communicate medication-related recommendations, contribute to treatment planning, and ensure continuity of care across different healthcare settings. This interdisciplinary collaboration enhances the quality and safety of medication therapy.

Documentation and Follow-Up: Clinical pharmacists document the outcomes of the medication therapy management interventions and develop care plans. They establish follow-up mechanisms to monitor the patient's progress, reassess medication regimens as needed, and provide ongoing support to address any medication-related issues that arise.

MTM services are typically provided to patients with complex medication regimens, multiple chronic conditions, or those at high risk for medication-related problems. MTM aims to improve medication outcomes, enhance patient satisfaction, reduce healthcare costs associated with medication-related issues, and promote optimal patient care.

By providing comprehensive medication management and patient-centered care, clinical pharmacists contribute to improved medication safety, adherence, and overall health outcomes. MTM services have resulted in better medication utilization, reduced hospital admissions, and improved patient quality of life.

3.2 Pharmaceutical Care

Traditional clinical pharmacy practices and pharmaceutical care are closely related and often overlap in their goals and approaches. While conventional clinical pharmacy practices focus on optimizing medication therapy and ensuring patient safety, pharmaceutical care takes it a step further by adopting a patient-centered approach and emphasizing the pharmacist's role in direct patient care. Let's explore the relationship between these two concepts in more detail:

Traditional clinical pharmacy practices include activities such as medication review and assessment, medication monitoring, medication education and counseling, medication safety, collaboration with healthcare teams, and adherence support. These practices aim to optimize medication therapy, improve patient outcomes, and ensure medication safety.

Pharmaceutical care builds upon traditional clinical pharmacy practices and adds the following elements:

Patient-Centered Approach: Pharmaceutical care places the patient at the center of the healthcare process. It focuses on understanding the patient's individual needs, preferences, and health goals. Clinical pharmacists engage in active communication and collaboration with patients to develop personalized care plans and establish therapeutic goals based on their specific needs.

Comprehensive Patient Assessment: Pharmaceutical care involves a comprehensive assessment of the patient, taking into account medical history, current medications, allergies, lifestyle factors, and individual preferences. This assessment helps identify potential medication-related issues and informs the development of individualized care plans.

Therapeutic Goal Setting: Pharmaceutical care emphasizes establishing mutually agreed-upon therapeutic goals between the clinical pharmacist and the patient. These goals align with the patient's health needs, values, and treatment outcomes. The plans go beyond symptom management and focus on disease control, prevention of medication-related problems, and improvement in overall quality of life.

Medication Optimization: Pharmaceutical care ensures the medication regimen is optimized for each patient. Clinical pharmacists review the medications for appropriateness, effectiveness, and safety. They consider factors such as drug interactions, duplications, contraindications, and the patient's characteristics. Clinical pharmacists collaborate with healthcare teams to make necessary adjustments to medication therapy to achieve optimal outcomes.

Patient Education and Counseling: Pharmaceutical care strongly emphasizes patient education and counseling. Clinical pharmacists provide comprehensive medication education, explaining the purpose of medications, proper administration, potential side effects, and precautions. They address patient concerns, answer questions, and empower patients to actively participate in their medication management and self-care.

Medication Adherence Support: Pharmaceutical care recognizes the importance of medication adherence in achieving optimal therapeutic outcomes. Clinical pharmacists assess barriers to adherence, work with patients to overcome challenges, and develop strategies to enhance medication adherence. They utilize adherence aids, reminder systems, and personalized adherence plans to support patients in sticking to their medication regimens.

Monitoring and Follow-up: Pharmaceutical care includes ongoing monitoring of patient's progress and medication therapy outcomes. Clinical pharmacists assess treatment effectiveness, evaluate for adverse effects or toxicities, and make necessary adjustments to optimize therapy. They establish follow-up mechanisms to ensure regular monitoring, address emerging medication-related issues, and support continuity of care.

Collaboration and Communication: Pharmaceutical care emphasizes collaboration and communication with other healthcare professionals involved in the patient's care. Clinical pharmacists actively participate in interdisciplinary rounds, contribute to treatment planning, and provide medication-related expertise to ensure coordinated and comprehensive patient care. This collaboration helps optimize medication therapy and enhances patient outcomes.

Pharmaceutical care expands on traditional clinical pharmacy practices by adopting a patient-centered approach, engaging in comprehensive patient assessments, setting therapeutic goals, optimizing medication therapy, providing extensive patient education and counseling, and offering adherence support. It emphasizes the importance of individualized care plans, patient empowerment, and ongoing monitoring to achieve optimal medication therapy outcomes and improve patient well-being.

3.3 Drug Information Services

Drug information services are an integral part of traditional clinical pharmacy practices. These services involve the provision of accurate, evidence-based, and up-to-date information on medications to healthcare professionals, patients, and other stakeholders. Drug information services aim to support informed decision-making regarding medication therapy, promote medication safety, and enhance patient care. Here are key aspects of drug information services within traditional clinical pharmacy practices:

Comprehensive Drug Knowledge: Clinical pharmacists possess in-depth knowledge of medications, including their pharmacology, indications, contraindications, dosages, interactions, adverse effects, and monitoring parameters. They stay updated with the latest research, clinical guidelines, and regulatory information related to medications.

Evidence-Based Drug Information: Clinical pharmacists critically evaluate the available evidence and provide evidence-based drug information. They review scientific literature, clinical trials, and other credible sources to ensure the information they provide is based on the best available evidence. This helps healthcare professionals make informed decisions regarding medication therapy.

Answering Drug-Related Inquiries: Clinical pharmacists respond to drug-related inquiries from healthcare professionals, including physicians, nurses, pharmacists, and other members of the healthcare team. They provide information on drug interactions, dosage adjustments, medication alternatives, adverse effects, compatibility, and other drug-related topics. These inquiries can be related to specific patients, drug therapies, or general medication inquiries.

Formulary Management: Clinical pharmacists play a role in formulary management within healthcare institutions. They evaluate medications for inclusion in the formulary based on their safety, efficacy, cost-effectiveness, and therapeutic value. Clinical pharmacists provide information to guide formulary decision-making and ensure the availability of appropriate and cost-effective medications.

Medication Safety: Clinical pharmacists contribute to medication safety by providing drug information to support safe medication use. They alert healthcare professionals to potential medication errors, adverse drug reactions, drug interactions, and medication-related risks. Clinical pharmacists assist in minimizing medication errors and promoting the safe use of medications.

Patient Counseling Support: Clinical pharmacists provide drug information and counseling to patients. They explain medication usage, potential side effects, precautions, and medication adherence strategies. Clinical pharmacists help patients make informed decisions about their medications, address their concerns, and empower them to participate in their own healthcare actively.

Medication Use Policies and Guidelines: Clinical pharmacists contribute to the development and implementation of medication use policies and guidelines within healthcare institutions. They provide input on medication-related protocols, dosing guidelines, therapeutic interchangeability, and medication-related policies to ensure safe and effective medication practices.

Continuing Education: Clinical pharmacists engage in continuous professional development and provide drug information updates to healthcare professionals. They conduct educational sessions, seminars, and in-service training on medication-related topics, ensuring healthcare professionals stay informed about new medications, guidelines, and emerging research.

Drug information services are essential in clinical pharmacy practices to ensure accurate and timely access to reliable drug information. These services support evidence-based decision-making, enhance patient safety, promote optimal medication therapy, and contribute to the overall quality of patient care. Clinical pharmacists play a critical role in improving medication knowledge, promoting medication safety, and optimizing medication therapy outcomes by providing drug information services.

3.4 Clinical Decision Support Systems

Clinical decision support systems (CDSS) are integral to traditional clinical pharmacy practices. CDSS are computer-based tools that assist healthcare professionals, including clinical pharmacists, make informed decisions regarding patient care and medication therapy. These systems provide evidence-based recommendations, alerts, and guidance to support clinical decision-making. Here are key aspects of clinical decision support systems within traditional clinical pharmacy practices:

Drug-Drug Interaction Checking: CDSS can automatically detect potential drug-drug interactions by comparing the patient's medication profile against a comprehensive database of known interactions. Clinical pharmacists can receive alerts and recommendations regarding the severity and management of identified interactions, allowing them to intervene and adjust the medication regimen appropriately.

Allergy and Adverse Reaction Alerts: CDSS can generate alerts when a patient has a known allergy or previous adverse reaction to a medication. Clinical pharmacists can review these alerts and take necessary precautions, such as recommending alternative medicines or implementing additional monitoring to prevent adverse events.

Medication Dosage Recommendations: CDSS can provide dosing recommendations based on patient-specific factors, such as age, weight, renal function, and comorbidities. Clinical pharmacists can utilize these recommendations to ensure that medications are prescribed at appropriate doses, reducing the risk of underdosing or overdosing.

Clinical Guidelines and Protocols: CDSS can integrate clinical guidelines and protocols into decision-making. By utilizing evidence-based guidelines, CDSS can provide recommendations for medication selection, dosing, and monitoring based on the patient's condition, improving the consistency and quality of care.

Drug Formulary Information: CDSS can incorporate information about the healthcare institution's drug formulary, including formulary status, preferred medications, and restrictions. Clinical pharmacists can use this information to ensure that prescribed medications are consistent with formulary guidelines and help guide appropriate medication selection.

Renal and Hepatic Dosing Support: CDSS can recommend medication dosing adjustments in patients with renal or hepatic impairment. This helps clinical pharmacists determine appropriate medication doses, reducing the risk of adverse effects or therapeutic failure in patients with impaired organ function.

Clinical Alerts and Reminders: CDSS can generate clinical alerts and reminders for various purposes, such as medication monitoring, laboratory test monitoring, and preventive care measures. These alerts prompt clinical pharmacists to take necessary actions, such as ordering laboratory tests or conducting follow-up assessments, to ensure ongoing patient safety and appropriate medication management.

Evidence-Based Decision Support: CDSS incorporates the latest evidence from clinical research, systematic reviews, and practice guidelines. This evidence-based approach supports clinical pharmacists in making informed decisions regarding medication therapy, ensuring that interventions align with current best practices and optimizing patient outcomes.

Clinical decision support systems enhance traditional clinical pharmacy practices by providing timely and evidence-based recommendations, alerts, and guidance to support medication management and patient care. They assist clinical pharmacists in identifying potential medication-related issues, reducing medication errors, improving medication safety, and optimizing medication therapy outcomes. By leveraging CDSS, clinical pharmacists can enhance their decision-making process, improve patient care, and contribute to improved patient outcomes.

3.5 Medication Reconciliation

Medication reconciliation is a critical component of traditional clinical pharmacy practices. It is a systematic process that involves comparing a patient's current medication regimen to all prescribed medications, including those from different healthcare settings or transitions of care. Medication reconciliation aims to identify discrepancies, resolve any medication-related issues, and ensure accurate and comprehensive medication information for safe and effective medication management. Here are key aspects of medication reconciliation within traditional clinical pharmacy practices:

Collection of Medication Information: Clinical pharmacists collect accurate and up-to-date information about a patient's medications from various sources, including the patient, healthcare providers, electronic health records, community pharmacies, and medication lists from previous encounters. This comprehensive medication history serves as a basis for conducting the reconciliation process.

Comparison and Identification of Discrepancies: Clinical pharmacists compare the patient's current medication regimen with the collected medication information to identify any discrepancies or differences. Distinctions can include omissions, duplications, incorrect dosages, drug interactions, and discrepancies in medication names or formulations.

Communication and Collaboration: Clinical pharmacists collaborate with other healthcare providers, including physicians, nurses, and pharmacists, to address identified discrepancies and resolve medication-related issues. They communicate any identified discrepancies, medication changes, and recommendations for medication management to ensure accurate and up-to-date medication records across the healthcare team.

Evaluation and Documentation: Clinical pharmacists evaluate the clinical significance of identified discrepancies and prioritize their resolution based on potential harm or impact on patient care. They document the reconciliation process, including the identified discrepancies, actions taken to resolve them, and any recommendations for ongoing medication management.

Medication Reconciliation at Transitions of Care: Medication reconciliation is particularly crucial during transitions of care, such as hospital admission, discharge, or transfer between healthcare facilities. Clinical pharmacists play an active role in ensuring that medication lists are accurately transferred between settings, reconciling medication changes, and facilitating continuity of care.

Patient Education and Counseling: Clinical pharmacists provide patient education and counseling regarding their medications as part of medication reconciliation. They explain any changes in the medication regimen, address discrepancies, and ensure that patients understand their medications, including proper usage, potential side effects, and adherence strategies.

Mediation of Medication Discrepancies: Clinical pharmacists take necessary actions to resolve identified discrepancies and medication-related issues. This may involve contacting prescribers to clarify medication orders, adjusting doses, discontinuing unnecessary medications, addressing potential drug interactions, and updating medication records.

Medication Safety and Continuity of Care: Medication reconciliation contributes to medication safety and continuity of care by ensuring accurate medication information across healthcare settings. It helps prevent medication errors, adverse drug events, and potential gaps in medication therapy during transitions or changes in care settings.

By incorporating medication reconciliation into their practice, clinical pharmacists play a vital role in promoting medication safety, reducing medication discrepancies, and ensuring accurate medication information. Medication reconciliation supports effective medication management, improves patient outcomes, and enhances the overall quality and continuity of care across different healthcare settings.

4. Technological Advances in Clinical Pharmacy

Dr. Rajesh Hadia

4.1 Electronic Health Records

Electronic Health Records (EHR) is a significant technological advancement in clinical pharmacy. EHRs are digital versions of patients' medical records that contain comprehensive and integrated health information, including medication profiles, medical history, laboratory results, diagnostic imaging, and other relevant data. Here are critical aspects of how electronic health records have transformed clinical pharmacy:

Centralized Medication Information: EHRs provide clinical pharmacists with centralized access to comprehensive medication information for individual patients. They can review medication histories, dosages, administration instructions, allergies, and previous adverse reactions, allowing for a more thorough medication therapy assessment.

Real-Time Medication Data: EHRs offer real-time updates on medication orders, dispensed medications, and medication administration records. This enables clinical pharmacists to access the most current patient medication regimen information, facilitating accurate medication review, monitoring, and reconciliation.

Medication Decision Support: EHRs integrate clinical decision support systems (CDSS) that provide alerts, reminders, and recommendations related to medication therapy. Clinical pharmacists can receive alerts for potential drug interactions, allergies, dosage adjustments, and adherence issues. These decision-support tools enhance medication safety, optimize medication selection, and aid in preventing medication-related errors.

Enhanced Medication Reconciliation: EHRs streamline the medication reconciliation by consolidating medication information from various sources. Clinical pharmacists can easily compare a patient's current medication regimen with historical data, facilitating identifying and resolving medication discrepancies during care transitions.

Facilitated Communication and Collaboration: EHRs enable seamless communication and collaboration among healthcare providers involved in patient care. Clinical pharmacists can securely share medication-related information, recommendations, and documentation with other healthcare team members, promoting efficient interdisciplinary collaboration and ensuring continuity of care.

Integration of Clinical Pharmacy Services: EHRs facilitate the integration of clinical pharmacy services within the healthcare system. Clinical pharmacists can document interventions, recommendations, and medication-related outcomes directly within the electronic health record, allowing for efficient communication and tracking of their contributions to patient care.

Medication Monitoring and Adherence: EHRs support medication monitoring and adherence by collecting and analyzing medication-related data. Clinical pharmacists can access information on medication refills, adherence patterns, and laboratory results to assess treatment effectiveness and intervene when necessary to optimize therapy and improve patient outcomes.

Data Analytics and Population Health Management: EHRs provide opportunities for data analytics and population health management initiatives. Clinical pharmacists can utilize aggregated data from

EHRs to identify medication trends, evaluate medication utilization patterns, and develop strategies for population-level interventions to enhance medication safety and effectiveness.

Research and Quality Improvement: EHRs offer a rich data source for research and quality improvement initiatives. Clinical pharmacists can leverage EHR data to conduct medication-related studies, evaluate outcomes of specific interventions, and contribute to evidence-based practice and quality improvement efforts in clinical pharmacy.

Electronic health records have revolutionized clinical pharmacy by improving access to comprehensive patient information, facilitating medication management processes, enhancing communication and collaboration, and providing decision support tools. Integrating EHRs into clinical pharmacy practice has resulted in more efficient and effective medication management, improved patient safety, and enhanced overall quality of care.

4.2 Telepharmacy

Telepharmacy is a significant technological advance in clinical pharmacy that allows pharmacists to provide pharmaceutical care remotely through telecommunication technology. It involves the delivery of pharmacy services, including medication counseling, prescription verification, and medication management, using audio and video conferencing, secure messaging, and other virtual communication tools. Here are critical aspects of how telepharmacy has transformed clinical pharmacy:

Remote Medication Dispensing: Telepharmacy enables pharmacists to remotely verify and dispense medications to patients located in underserved or remote areas. Through secure electronic systems, pharmacists can review prescriptions, verify medication orders, and remotely supervise dispensing, ensuring that patients have access to necessary medications.

Medication Counseling and Education: Telepharmacy allows pharmacists to provide medication counseling and education remotely. Pharmacists can conduct video or audio consultations with patients, address medication-related questions, provide instructions on medication use, explain potential side effects, and promote medication adherence. Telepharmacy enhances patient access to medication information and enables pharmacists to reach patients who may have limited physical access to healthcare facilities.

Medication Therapy Management (MTM): Telepharmacy facilitates the provision of MTM services remotely. Pharmacists can review medication regimens, conduct comprehensive medication reviews, assess medication adherence, and make recommendations for therapy optimization, all through virtual communication platforms. Telepharmacy expands the reach of MTM services, allowing pharmacists to provide care to patients who may not have easy access to in-person consultations.

Medication Reconciliation and Transitions of Care: Telepharmacy supports medication reconciliation during transitions of care, such as hospital discharge or transfers between healthcare settings. Pharmacists can remotely review medication lists, verify accuracy, resolve discrepancies, and ensure continuity of care. Telepharmacy enables timely reconciliation, reducing the risk of medication errors and improving patient safety.

Medication Adherence Support: Telepharmacy plays a crucial role in promoting medication adherence. Pharmacists can remotely assess medication adherence, identify barriers, and develop strategies to enhance patient adherence, such as reminder systems, medication packaging solutions, and adherence counseling. Through virtual communication, pharmacists can provide ongoing support and monitoring to improve patient adherence.

Collaborative Care and Interprofessional Communication: Telepharmacy facilitates collaboration among healthcare professionals, allowing pharmacists to participate in interdisciplinary rounds, case discussions, and consultations remotely. Virtual communication platforms enable seamless and secure communication between pharmacists, physicians, nurses, and other members of the healthcare team, ensuring effective interprofessional communication and coordinated patient care.

Remote Medication Monitoring: Telepharmacy enables pharmacists to remotely monitor patient response to medication therapy. Through telecommunication tools, pharmacists can review laboratory results, assess medication efficacy, evaluate for adverse effects, and make appropriate adjustments to medication regimens. Remote monitoring enhances patient care and allows for timely interventions when necessary.

Medication Safety and Adverse Event Prevention: Telepharmacy supports medication safety through the remote review of medication orders, identification of potential drug interactions or adverse effects, and verification of medication appropriateness. Pharmacists can provide real-time recommendations to prevent medication-related errors and adverse events, improving patient safety.

Telepharmacy has transformed clinical pharmacy by overcoming geographical barriers, improving access to pharmaceutical care, enhancing patient education and counseling, promoting medication adherence, and facilitating interprofessional collaboration. It has proven particularly valuable in underserved areas, remote regions, and situations where in-person consultations may be challenging. Telepharmacy expands the reach of clinical pharmacy services, improves patient outcomes, and enhances the overall quality of care.

4.3 Clinical Pharmacy Software

Clinical pharmacy software refers to computer-based applications and platforms designed specifically for clinical pharmacy practice. These software solutions offer various functionalities to support medication management, patient care, documentation, communication, and decision-making. Here are key aspects of how clinical pharmacy software has advanced the field:

Medication Management: Clinical pharmacy software provides tools for medication management, including electronic prescribing, medication order entry, and medication dispensing systems. These systems enhance accuracy, efficiency, and safety by minimizing medication errors, automating order processing, and supporting clinical decision-making.

Clinical Decision Support: Clinical pharmacy software integrates clinical decision support systems (CDSS) that provide alerts, reminders, and recommendations related to medication therapy. CDSS within the software offers real-time guidance based on evidence-based guidelines, medication interactions, dosage adjustments, and patient-specific factors. This helps clinical pharmacists make informed decisions and optimize medication therapy.

Medication Reconciliation: Clinical pharmacy software incorporates medication reconciliation modules that facilitate the process of comparing a patient's current medication regimen with medication history, identifying discrepancies, and documenting changes. This streamlines medication reconciliation during transitions of care, reducing errors and ensuring accurate medication information.

Electronic Health Records Integration: Clinical pharmacy software integrates with electronic health record (EHR) systems, allowing seamless access to comprehensive patient information. This integration enables clinical pharmacists to review medication histories, laboratory results, diagnostic reports, and other relevant patient data, enhancing medication management and decision-making.

Documentation and Reporting: Clinical pharmacy software provides robust documentation and reporting features. Pharmacists can efficiently document interventions, medication-related assessments, care plans, and outcomes within the software. These documentation capabilities facilitate communication, track interventions, and support quality improvement initiatives.

Adverse Drug Event Monitoring: Clinical pharmacy software incorporates modules for adverse drug event monitoring and reporting. Pharmacists can enter and track adverse drug events, analyze trends, and generate reports for analysis and further investigation. This functionality helps in detecting and preventing medication-related harm.

Communication and Collaboration: Clinical pharmacy software includes communication and collaboration features to facilitate interdisciplinary teamwork and communication among healthcare professionals. Pharmacists can securely communicate with physicians, nurses, and other members of the healthcare team, share information, and collaborate on patient care through messaging systems and task management tools.

Data Analytics and Clinical Insights: Clinical pharmacy software offers analytics capabilities that enable pharmacists to analyze medication-related data, identify trends, and generate reports for research, quality improvement initiatives, and population health management. These insights support evidence-based practice and enhance patient care.

Patient Engagement and Education: Clinical pharmacy software may include patient portals or interfaces that allow patients to access medication information, receive educational materials, and communicate with pharmacists. This promotes patient engagement, medication adherence, and patient-centered care.

Clinical pharmacy software has revolutionized clinical pharmacy practice by streamlining medication management, enhancing medication safety, supporting clinical decision-making, improving documentation and communication, and facilitating data-driven insights. These software solutions have become essential tools for clinical pharmacists, enabling them to deliver efficient, evidence-based, and pat-centered care.

4.4 Pharmacy Automation Systems

Pharmacy automation systems are technological advancements that have significantly impacted clinical pharmacy practice. These systems automate various tasks involved in medication dispensing, inventory management, and prescription processing, enhancing efficiency, accuracy, and patient safety. Here are key aspects of how pharmacy automation systems have transformed clinical pharmacy:

Medication Dispensing: Pharmacy automation systems automate the process of medication dispensing. Robotic dispensing systems can accurately count, package, and label medications, reducing the risk of dispensing errors and improving efficiency. Automated dispensing cabinets (ADCs) are used in healthcare facilities to store and dispense medications, ensuring secure and controlled access to medicines for healthcare providers.

Prescription Processing: Pharmacy automation systems streamline prescription processing by automating prescription order entry, verification, and label printing tasks. These systems integrate with electronic health record (EHR) systems and allow for seamless transfer of prescription information, reducing manual data entry errors and improving workflow efficiency.

Medication Packaging: Pharmacy automation systems offer medication packaging solutions, such as unit-dose packaging or multi-dose blister packs. These packaging systems help improve medication adherence by organizing medications by dose and administration time. They also assist in reducing medication errors and simplifying medication administration for patients and healthcare providers.

Barcode Scanning and Verification: Pharmacy automation systems incorporate barcode scanning technology to verify medication accuracy. Barcode scanners can match the medication barcode with the prescription information, ensuring the correct medication is dispensed. This verification process reduces the risk of medication errors and enhances patient safety.

Inventory Management: Pharmacy automation systems assist with inventory management by tracking medication stock levels, expiration dates, and reorder points. These systems can automatically generate inventory reports, facilitate medication stock rotation, and streamline ordering. This helps optimize medication inventory, reduce waste, and ensure medication availability.

Medication Safety Checks: Pharmacy automation systems include safety checks and verification processes to prevent medication errors. These systems use technology such as barcode scanning, image recognition, and electronic verification to ensure the accuracy of medication selection and reduce the risk of dispensing the wrong medication or dosage.

Documentation and Reporting: Pharmacy automation systems provide documentation and reporting capabilities, allowing pharmacists to track and document medication-related activities. These systems generate reports on dispensing accuracy, inventory usage, medication reconciliation, and other metrics, aiding in quality improvement efforts and regulatory compliance.

Workflow Efficiency: Pharmacy automation systems improve workflow efficiency by automating time-consuming tasks, reducing manual labor, and minimizing the potential for human error. This enables pharmacists to focus more on patient care activities, medication counseling, and clinical decision-making.

Integration with Clinical Pharmacy Services: Pharmacy automation systems can be integrated with clinical decision support systems (CDSS) and electronic health record (EHR) systems, enabling seamless communication and access to patient information. This integration enhances medication management, clinical decision-making, and interprofessional collaboration.

Pharmacy automation systems have revolutionized medication dispensing, inventory management, and prescription processing in clinical pharmacy. They improve medication safety, accuracy, workflow efficiency, and patient care. By automating routine tasks, these systems free up clinical pharmacists' time to focus on direct patient care, medication counseling, and clinical interventions, ultimately enhancing the overall quality of pharmacy services.

4.5 Mobile Applications in Clinical Pharmacy

Mobile applications have become valuable tools in clinical pharmacy, offering convenient access to information, resources, and tools that support medication management, patient care, and professional development. Here are critical aspects of how mobile applications have advanced clinical pharmacy:

Medication Information and References: Mobile applications provide access to comprehensive drug databases, medication references, and formularies. Clinical pharmacists can quickly search for drug information, including dosing guidelines, interactions, adverse effects, and pharmacokinetics, enhancing their knowledge base and facilitating evidence-based decision-making.

Clinical Decision Support: Mobile applications incorporate clinical decision support tools that offer real-time guidance and recommendations based on patient-specific factors and evidence-based guidelines. These tools provide alerts for potential drug interactions, dosage adjustments, and medication safety considerations, aiding in medication selection and optimization.

Medication Adherence Support: Mobile applications offer features to support medication adherence. These applications can send reminders for medication administration, track compliance through medication log entries, and provide educational materials and resources to improve patient understanding andcommitmente.

Telehealth and Remote Consultations: Mobile applications enable telehealth consultations and remote patient monitoring. Clinical pharmacists can use video conferencing or secure messaging to communicate with patients, conduct medication counseling sessions, and provide follow-up care, extending their reach beyond traditional healthcare settings.

Medication Reconciliation: Mobile applications facilitate medication reconciliation during transitions of care. Pharmacists can use these applications to compare medication lists, identify discrepancies, and make necessary updates. Mobile applications streamline the reconciliation process and improve accuracy and communication among healthcare providers.

Continuing Education and Professional Development: Mobile applications offer access to continuing education resources, pharmaceutical journals, research articles, and clinical updates. Clinical pharmacists can stay updated with the latest advancements, guidelines, and research in their field, supporting their professional development.

Medication Safety and Reporting: Mobile applications provide platforms for reporting adverse drug reactions, medication errors, and safety incidents. Clinical pharmacists can document and report incidents directly through the application, contributing to medication safety surveillance and quality improvement efforts.

Collaboration and Communication: Mobile applications facilitate cooperation and communication among healthcare providers. Pharmacists can securely communicate with physicians, nurses, and other team members, exchange information, and seek consultation on patient cases, promoting coordinated and patient-centered care.

Patient Education and Resources: Mobile applications offer patient education materials, medication guides, and resources to share with patients. Clinical pharmacists can use these tools to enhance patient understanding, promote self-management, and provide reliable information to support shared decision-making.

Mobile applications in clinical pharmacies leverage the convenience and ubiquity of smartphones to enhance medication management, patient care, and professional development. These applications provide pharmacists with accessible resources, decision support tools, communication platforms, and patient engagement solutions. By utilizing mobile applications, clinical pharmacists can improve efficiency, enhance medication safety, and provide patients with more personalized and convenient care.

5. Precision Medicine and Personalized Pharmacotherapy

Dr. Rajesh Hadia

5.1 Genomics and Pharmacogenomics

Precision medicine and personalized pharmacotherapy aim to tailor medical treatment and medication choices to individual patients based on their unique characteristics. Genomics and pharmacogenomics play crucial roles in these approaches. Let's explore the concepts of genomics and pharmacogenomics within the context of precision medicine and personalized pharmacotherapy:

Genomics:

Genomics is the study of an individual's entire genome, which comprises all the genes and DNA sequences within their cells. Advances in genomics have provided insights into the genetic variations and variations in gene expression that can influence an individual's response to medications.

Pharmacogenomics:

Pharmacogenomics focuses on how an individual's genetic makeup influences their medication response. It involves studying how genetic variations affect drug metabolism, drug targets, andtargets; Pharmacogenomic information can help predict how an individual will respond to specific medications, enabling personalized medication selection and dosing.

Benefits of Genomics and Pharmacogenomics in Precision Medicine and Personalized Pharmacotherapy:

Personalized Medication Selection: Genomic and pharmacogenomic information can assist healthcare providers in selecting the most appropriate medication for an individual based on their genetic profile. By considering an individual's genetic variations, healthcare providers can identify drugs that are likely to be effective and avoid those that may be less effective or cause adverse reactions.

Optimal Medication Dosing: Genetic variations can impact the way medications are metabolized and cleared from the body. Pharmacogenomic information helps determine the optimal medication dosage for an individual, taking into account the genetic factors that influence drug metabolism. This precision dosing reduces the risk of under- or overdosing and improves medication efficacy and safety.

Predicting Adverse Drug Reactions: Certain genetic variations can increase the risk of adverse drug reactions or drug toxicity. Pharmacogenomic testing can identify individuals who are at a higher risk, allowing healthcare providers to select alternative medications or adjust dosages to minimize the likelihood of adverse reactions.

Improved Treatment Outcomes: By tailoring medication choices and dosages to an individual's genetic profile, precision medicine and personalized pharmacotherapy have the potential to enhance treatment outcomes. Patients are more likely to respond positively to medications that are specifically selected and dosed based on their genetic characteristics, leading to improved efficacy and fewer adverse effects.

Avoidance of Ineffective Treatments: Genomic and pharmacogenomic information can help identify individuals who are unlikely to respond to certain medications. This information allows healthcare providers to avoid prescribing medications that are unlikely to be effective, saving patients from unnecessary treatments and associated side effects.

Reduction in Trial-and-Error Approach: Traditional medication prescribing often involves a trial-and-error approach, where patients may need to try multiple medications before finding one that works for them. By integrating genomics and pharmacogenomics, healthcare providers can reduce the trial-and-error process and prescribe medications more effectively and efficiently.

Challenges:

Despite the potential benefits, there are challenges associated with the integration of genomics and pharmacogenomics into clinical practice. These challenges include the interpretation of genetic data, the availability of comprehensive genomic databases, the need for specialized training among healthcare providers, ethical considerations related to genetic testing, and the cost and accessibility of genomic testing.

Genomics and pharmacogenomics are transforming clinical practice by enabling personalized pharmacotherapy and precision medicine. These approaches allow healthcare providers to tailor medication choices and dosages to individual patients based on their genetic characteristics, ultimately leading to improved treatment outcomes, reduced adverse reactions, and optimized medication efficacy.

5.2 Biomarkers in Clinical Decision Making

Biomarkers play a critical role in clinical decision-making in precision medicine and personalized pharmacotherapy. Biomarkers are measurable indicators, such as molecules or genetic markers, that can provide information about a patient's health status, disease progression, or response to treatment. By analyzing biomarkers, healthcare providers can make informed decisions regarding medication selection, treatment strategies, and monitoring. Here are key aspects of the use of biomarkers in clinical decision-making:

Disease Diagnosis and Subtyping: Biomarkers can aid in the diagnosis and subtyping of diseases. They can help differentiate between different disease subtypes or stages, leading to more precise diagnoses and tailored treatment approaches. For example, biomarkers may be used to identify specific genetic mutations in cancer cells to guide targeted therapies.

Predicting Treatment Response: Biomarkers can provide insight into an individual's likelihood of responding to a particular medication or treatment. By analyzing specific biomarkers, healthcare providers can predict treatment outcomes and select the most effective treatment options for patients. This helps avoid unnecessary treatments and minimizes the risk of adverse effects.

Treatment Monitoring: Biomarkers can be used to monitor the response to treatment and assess treatment effectiveness over time. By measuring biomarkers during the course of therapy, healthcare providers can evaluate treatment response, make adjustments as needed, and determine if treatment modifications or alternative therapies are necessary.

Individualized Dosing: Biomarkers can guide individualized dosing strategies. Some biomarkers, such as drug-metabolizing enzymes or genetic variations, can influence how a patient's body processes medications. By considering these biomarkers, healthcare providers can personalize medication dosing to optimize therapeutic outcomes and minimize the risk of adverse reactions.

Prognostic Assessment: Biomarkers can provide prognostic information, helping predict the likely course of a disease and the expected outcomes for an individual patient. This information can guide treatment decisions and help healthcare providers and patients make informed choices regarding treatment strategies, goals, and follow-up care.

Risk Stratification: Biomarkers can assist in risk stratification, identifying individuals who are at higher risk for disease development, disease progression, or adverse events. By analyzing specific biomarkers, healthcare providers can identify high-risk patients and implement preventive measures, early interventions, or intensified monitoring to mitigate risks and improve patient outcomes.

Therapeutic Drug Monitoring: Biomarkers can guide therapeutic drug monitoring, where medication levels in the body are measured to ensure optimal dosing and avoid toxicity. Biomarkers, such as drug concentrations in blood or specific metabolites, can help healthcare providers tailor medication dosing based on individual variability, optimizing treatment efficacy and safety.

Clinical Trial Selection: Biomarkers can assist in patient selection for clinical trials. By identifying individuals who possess specific biomarkers associated with a targeted therapy or treatment response, clinical trials can enroll patients who are more likely to benefit from the intervention, improving the efficiency and success rate of clinical trials.

The use of biomarkers in clinical decision-making allows for a more personalized and targeted approach to patient care. By integrating biomarkers into clinical practice, healthcare providers can select the most appropriate treatments, individualize medication dosing, monitor treatment response, and predict patient outcomes. This promotes precision medicine, enhances treatment efficacy, minimizes adverse events, and ultimately improves patient outcomes.

5.3 Individualized Treatment Approaches

Individualized treatment approaches are a key aspect of precision medicine and personalized pharmacotherapy. These approaches aim to tailor medical treatments and medication choices to individual patients based on their unique characteristics, including genetic makeup, biomarker profiles, clinical features, and lifestyle factors. Here are key aspects of individualized treatment approaches:

Genetic Variations: Genetic information plays a crucial role in individualized treatment approaches. By analyzing a patient's genetic variations, healthcare providers can identify specific genetic markers associated with disease susceptibility, treatment response, and adverse reactions. This information helps guide medication selection, dosing, and treatment strategies.

Biomarker Analysis: Biomarkers, such as protein levels, gene expression patterns, or specific molecules, can provide valuable insights into a patient's disease status, prognosis, and response to treatment. By analyzing biomarkers, healthcare providers can personalize treatment decisions, monitor treatment response, and adjust therapies accordingly.

Disease Subtypes: Diseases often have multiple subtypes or variations, each requiring a tailored approach to treatment. By identifying specific disease subtypes through genetic testing, molecular profiling, or other diagnostic techniques, healthcare providers can customize treatment plans based on the unique characteristics of each subtype.

Pharmacogenomics: Pharmacogenomics involves studying how an individual's genetic makeup affects their response to medications. By considering pharmacogenomic information, healthcare providers can predict an individual's likelihood of responding to specific medications, determine optimal dosing, and avoid medications that may lead to adverse reactions.

Lifestyle Factors: Individualized treatment approaches take into account lifestyle factors that can influence treatment outcomes. Factors such as diet, exercise, smoking habits, and environmental exposures can impact a patient's response to treatment. By considering these factors, healthcare providers can integrate lifestyle modifications and personalized recommendations into the treatment plan.

Comorbidities and Co-medications: Individualized treatment approaches consider a patient's comorbidities (co-existing medical conditions) and co-medications (other medications the patient is taking). These factors can affect treatment choices, drug interactions, and potential adverse effects. Healthcare providers evaluate the individual's overall health status and tailor treatment plans accordingly.

Patient Preferences and Values: Individualized treatment approaches also take into account patient preferences, values, and goals. Shared decision-making between healthcare providers and patients allows for a collaborative approach to treatment planning, considering the patient's preferences, lifestyle, beliefs, and treatment goals.

Continuous Monitoring and Adaptation: Individualized treatment approaches involve constant monitoring and adaptation based on the patient's response to treatment. Regular assessments, biomarker monitoring, and patient feedback help healthcare providers track treatment efficacy and make necessary adjustments to optimize outcomes.

Healthcare providers can optimize treatment outcomes, minimize adverse reactions, and improve patient satisfaction by adopting individualized treatment approaches. These approaches move away from the one-size-fits-all approach and emphasize the importance of tailoring treatment plans to t each patient's unique characteristics and needs. Precision medicine and personalized pharmacotherapy pave the way for more targeted, effective, and patient-centered care.

5.4 Challenges and Opportunities

While precision medicine and personalized pharmacotherapy offer significant opportunities for improving patient care, some challenges need to be addressed. Here are some of the key challenges and opportunities associated with these approaches:

Challenges:

Data Integration and Interpretation: Precision medicine relies on the integration and analysis of large amounts of data, including genetic, clinical, and environmental information. The challenge lies in effectively integrating and interpreting these diverse data sources to derive meaningful insights for personalized treatment decisions.

Limited Access to Biomarker Testing: Availability and accessibility of biomarker testing can be a challenge. Some biomarker tests may be expensive, require specialized equipment or expertise, or be limited to specific healthcare settings. Ensuring widespread access to biomarker testing is essential for the successful implementation of personalized pharmacotherapy.

Ethical and Privacy Considerations: Precision medicine raises ethical concerns related to the use of genetic and personal health information. Safeguarding patient privacy, obtaining informed consent for genetic testing, and addressing potential discrimination or stigmatization based on genetic information are important ethical considerations that need to be addressed.

Cost and Reimbursement: The cost of implementing precision medicine approaches, including genetic testing, data analysis, and personalized treatment options, can be a significant barrier. Establishing reimbursement mechanisms and addressing cost-effectiveness are essential for the widespread adoption and accessibility of personalized pharmacotherapy.

Education and Training: Healthcare providers need to be adequately trained and educated in the principles and applications of precision medicine. Training programs should be developed to enhance healthcare professionals' knowledge and skills in interpreting genetic and biomarker data, understanding treatment implications, and effectively communicating personalized treatment options to patients.

Opportunities:

Improved Treatment Efficacy and Safety: Precision medicine and personalized pharmacotherapy have the potential to significantly improve treatment efficacy and safety by tailoring treatments to individual patient characteristics. By understanding genetic variations, biomarkers, and patient-specific factors, healthcare providers can optimize treatment decisions and minimize adverse effects.

Targeted Therapies and Reduced Trial-and-Error: Personalized pharmacotherapy enables the identification of targeted therapies that are most likely to be effective for individual patients. This reduces the need for a trial-and-error approach in treatment selection and leads to more efficient and effective treatment outcomes.

Prevention and Early Intervention: Precision medicine allows for early identification of individuals at risk of certain diseases or adverse drug reactions. This enables preventive measures, early intervention, and close monitoring to minimize disease progression and improve patient outcomes.

Advancements in Biomarker Research: Ongoing advancements in biomarker research, including the identification of novel biomarkers, provide opportunities for further refining personalized pharmacotherapy approaches. New biomarkers can enhance treatment selection, monitoring, and prediction of treatment response.

Collaboration and Data Sharing: Precision medicine requires collaboration and data sharing across healthcare institutions, research organizations, and industry partners. Collaborative efforts facilitate the accumulation of large datasets, leading to more robust research, improved understanding of disease mechanisms, and the development of targeted therapies.

Patient Empowerment and Engagement: Precision medicine promotes patient engagement and shared decision-making. Patients are empowered with information about their genetic and biomarker profiles, enabling them to actively participate in treatment decisions, understand potential risks and benefits, and contribute to their own personalized care plans.

Research and Innovation: Precision medicine opens up new avenues for research and innovation in pharmacogenomics, biomarker discovery, and targeted therapies. These advancements can lead to novel treatments, improvement of existing therapies, and advances in diagnostic tools.

Addressing the challenges and embracing the opportunities of precision medicine and personalized pharmacotherapy requires collaboration among healthcare professionals, policymakers, researchers, and industry stakeholders. By overcoming barriers and leveraging the potential of these approaches, clinical pharmacy can advance toward more personalized, effective, and patient-centered care.

6. Integration of Pharmacists in Interprofessional Healthcare Teams

Dr. Rajesh Hadia

6.1 Collaborative Practice Models

The integration of pharmacists in interprofessional healthcare teams has been recognized as a valuable approach to improving patient care and optimizing medication management. Collaborative practice models involve pharmacists working alongside other healthcare professionals, such as physicians, nurses, and allied health professionals, to deliver comprehensive and coordinated patient care. Here are some common collaborative practice models that involve pharmacists:

Multidisciplinary Teams: In this model, healthcare professionals from various disciplines, including pharmacists, work together to provide patient care. Each team member contributes their expertise, knowledge, and skills to develop and implement patient care plans. Pharmacists play a crucial role in medication management, providing medication-related expertise, and drug information, and contributing to medication therapy decision-making.

Interprofessional Collaborative Teams: Interprofessional collaborative teams involve healthcare professionals from different disciplines actively engaging in shared decision-making and collaborative practice. Pharmacists collaborate with other healthcare team members to discuss patient cases, develop treatment plans, and coordinate medication-related interventions. This model promotes communication, coordination, and a patient-centered approach to care.

Medication Therapy Management (MTM) Teams: MTM teams consist of pharmacists and other healthcare professionals who work together to optimize medication therapy for patients. Pharmacists play a central role in medication assessment, monitoring, and providing recommendations for medication optimization. Collaboration within the MTM team helps identify medication-related issues, develop care plans, and implement interventions to enhance patient outcomes.

Integrated Care Teams: Integrated care teams bring together healthcare professionals from different settings, such as hospitals, primary care clinics, and community pharmacies, to deliver coordinated care to patients across different healthcare settings. Pharmacists collaborate with other team members to ensure continuity of care, provide medication counseling, address medication-related issues, and promote medication adherence.

Transitions of Care Teams: Care teams focus on smooth patient transitions between different healthcare settings, such as hospitals, rehabilitation facilities, and home care. Pharmacists contribute to these teams by conducting medication reconciliation, ensuring accurate medication lists, providing patient education, and coordinating medication management during transitions.

Chronic Disease Management Teams: In established disease management teams, healthcare professionals collaborate to provide comprehensive care to patients with chronic conditions. Pharmacists play an integral role in medication management, conducting medication reviews, monitoring treatment efficacy, promoting adherence, and providing patient education on the appropriate use of medications.

These collaborative practice models recognize the expertise of pharmacists in medication management and the importance of their contributions to patient care. Integrating pharmacists into interprofessional healthcare teams can improve patient outcomes through enhanced medication safety, optimization, and patient education and adherence. Effective communication, shared decision-making, and a patient-centered approach are essential components of successful collaborative practice models.

6.2 Team-Based Care and Communication

Integrating pharmacists in interprofessional healthcare teams emphasizes the importance of team-based care and effective communication among team members. Here are critical aspects of team-based care and communication in the context of pharmacists' integration into interprofessional healthcare teams:

Shared Goals and Patient-Centered Care: Interprofessional teams work collaboratively to establish goals focused on providing patient-centered care. The team members, including pharmacists, align their efforts to ensure the best possible patient outcomes. The patient's needs, preferences, and values guide the decision-making process.

Clear Roles and Responsibilities: Each team member, including pharmacists, has clearly defined roles and responsibilities within the interprofessional team. This clarity helps avoid duplication of efforts, ensures that each team member contributes their expertise effectively, and enhances overall team efficiency.

Effective Communication: Communication is a cornerstone of successful interprofessional collaboration. Open and respectful communication among team members, including pharmacists, promotes shared understanding, coordination, and effective decision-making. Regular team meetings, huddles, and electronic communication platforms facilitate the timely exchange of information and updates.

Mutual Respect and Trust: Building a mutual respect and trust culture is essential for effective teamwork. Recognizing and valuing each team member's expertise, including pharmacists, fosters an environment of trust, psychological safety, and collaboration. Trust enables open dialogue, sharing of perspectives, and effective resolution of conflicts.

Collaborative Care Planning: Interprofessional teams, including pharmacists, collaborate in care planning, considering multiple perspectives and expertise. Pharmacists contribute knowledge of medication management, drug interactions, and patient-specific factors, ensuring that medication-related considerations are integrated into the care plan. Team members collectively establish treatment goals, develop care plans, and monitor patient progress.

Interdisciplinary Rounds: Interdisciplinary rounds bring together healthcare professionals, including pharmacists, to discuss patient cases, review medication regimens, and make collaborative decisions regarding treatment plans. These rounds promote comprehensive assessments, facilitate interdisciplinary communication, and ensure coordinated care.

Documentation and Information Sharing: Effective communication extends to documentation and information sharing. Accurate and timely documentation, including medication-related information, is vital for continuity of care. Electronic health records and communication systems facilitate secure and efficient information sharing among team members, ensuring that relevant information is accessible to all.

Continuous Learning and Professional Development: Interprofessional teams foster a culture of constant learning and professional development. Team members, including pharmacists, engage in ongoing education, attend team-based training, and share their knowledge and experiences. This collaborative learning environment enhances team effectiveness and promotes the delivery of evidence-based care.

Quality Improvement and Outcomes Measurement: Interprofessional teams work together to assess and improve the quality of care provided. Regular review of outcomes, performance indicators, and patient feedback allows the team, including pharmacists, to identify areas for improvement, implement evidence-based practices, and monitor progress toward achieving optimal patient outcomes.

By embracing team-based care and effective communication, interprofessional healthcare teams can harness the expertise of pharmacists and other professionals, leading to improved patient outcomes, enhanced medication management, and a patient-centered approach to care. Collaboration, communication, and a shared commitment to patient well-being are critical factors in successful interprofessional practice.

6.3 Improved Patient Outcomes

The integration of pharmacists in interprofessional healthcare teams has been shown to positively impact patient outcomes. By collaborating with other healthcare professionals, pharmacists contribute their expertise in medication management and play a vital role in improving patient care. Here are some ways in which the integration of pharmacists in interprofessional teams leads to improved patient outcomes:

Medication Optimization: Pharmacists play a crucial role in medication optimization by reviewing medication regimens, identifying potential drug interactions or adverse effects, and recommending appropriate adjustments. This helps ensure patients receive the most effective and safe medications tailored to their needs, leading to improved treatment outcomes.

Medication Adherence: Poor medication adherence is a common issue that can negatively impact treatment outcomes. As part of interprofessional teams, pharmacists can educate patients about their medications, provide counseling on proper usage, and address any concerns or barriers to adherence. Their involvement has been shown to improve medication adherence rates and, enhance treatment efficacy.

Medication Safety: Pharmacists are experts in medication safety, and their integration into interprofessional teams can significantly reduce medication errors and adverse drug events. Through medication reconciliation, comprehensive medication reviews, and ongoing monitoring, pharmacists help identify and prevent potential medication-related problems, ensuring patient safety.

Chronic Disease Management: Pharmacists contribute to chronic disease management by providing education, monitoring disease progression, and assisting with medication management. By working collaboratively with other healthcare professionals, pharmacists help patients better understand their conditions, adhere to treatment plans, and make lifestyle modifications, resulting in improved management of chronic diseases.

Preventive Care: As part of interprofessional teams, pharmacists can actively engage in preventive care efforts. They can provide immunizations, perform health screenings, and offer counseling on lifestyle modifications and risk reduction. This proactive approach contributes to early detection, prevention, and management of health conditions, leading to improved patient outcomes.

Transitions of Care: Transitions between healthcare settings, such as hospital to home or hospital to a long-term care facility, are critical and can be associated with medication-related issues. Pharmacists play a key role in ensuring smooth care transitions by conducting medication reconciliation, identifying and resolving discrepancies, and educating patients and caregivers. This reduces the risk of medication errors and adverse events during care transitions.

Interdisciplinary Collaboration: The integration of pharmacists in interprofessional teams promotes effective collaboration and communication among healthcare professionals. This collaborative approach facilitates the exchange of information, enhances coordinated care, and minimizes fragmentation. The seamless coordination among team members ensures that patients receive comprehensive, holistic care, leading to improved outcomes.

Patient Education and Empowerment: Pharmacists contribute to patient education, providing information about medications, potential side effects, and self-care strategies. By empowering patients with knowledge, promoting shared decision-making, and involving them in their treatment plans, pharmacists help patients take an active role in their healthcare, leading to better treatment adherence and outcomes.

Quality Improvement: Interprofessional teams, with pharmacists' involvement, engage in quality improvement initiatives. They analyze patient outcomes, identify areas for improvement, implement evidence-based practices, and monitor progress. This continuous quality improvement approach ensures that patient care is continually optimized, leading to better outcomes over time.

The integration of pharmacists in interprofessional healthcare teams has a positive impact on patient outcomes by improving medication management, promoting medication adherence, ensuring medication safety, enhancing chronic disease management, facilitating transitions of care, fostering interdisciplinary collaboration, empowering patients, and driving quality improvement efforts. This collaborative approach to patient care maximizes the expertise of each team member, leading to improved overall patient outcomes and healthcare delivery.

6.4 Barriers and Facilitators

The integration of pharmacists in interprofessional healthcare teams is essential for optimizing patient care. However, several barriers and facilitators can influence the successful implementation of this integration. Here are some common barriers and facilitators to consider:

Barriers:

Limited Awareness and Understanding: Some healthcare professionals may have little awareness of the role and scope of practice of pharmacists. A lack of understanding about the expertise and contributions of pharmacists can hinder their integration into interprofessional teams.

Fragmented Healthcare Systems: Fragmentation within healthcare systems, with limited collaboration and communication among healthcare professionals, can impede the integration of pharmacists into interprofessional teams. Siloed practices and a lack of standardized processes may hinder effective collaboration.

Organizational Structures and Policies: Organizational structures and policies may only sometimes support the integration of pharmacists into interprofessional teams. Hierarchical structures, restrictive policies, and a lack of incentives for collaboration can create barriers to effective teamwork.

Time and Workload Constraints: Healthcare professionals often face time constraints and heavy workloads, which can limit collaboration and interdisciplinary communication opportunities. The lack of dedicated time for interprofessional collaboration can make it challenging for pharmacists to a to participate in team-based care actively *ofessional Identity and Autonomy:* Professional identity and autonomy can influence the willingness of healthcare professionals, including pharmacists, to collaborate. Healthcare professionals may have concerns about relinquishing control over certain aspects of patient care or may be resistant to integrating the expertise of other professionals into their practice.

Communication and Information-Sharing Challenges: Inadequate communication and information-sharing systems can hinder effective collaboration. Access to shared electronic health records, efficient communication platforms, or lack of standardized communication protocols may create barriers to seamless information exchange among team members.

Facilitators:

Interprofessional Education and Training: Providing interprofessional education and training during healthcare professionals' formative years can promote a better understanding of each profession's role and foster a collaborative mindset. Exposure to interprofessional learning environments helps build the foundation for effective teamwork.

Clear Roles and Responsibilities: Clearly defining and communicating the roles and responsibilities of each team member, including pharmacists, promotes efficient teamwork. Understanding each other's expertise and contributions fosters respect and appreciation for the unique skills that each profession brings to the team.

Supportive Organizational Culture: An organizational culture that values interprofessional collaboration and team-based care is crucial. Supportive policies, structures, and leadership that encourage interdisciplinary communication shared decision-making, and collaborative practice facilitate the integration of pharmacists into interprofessional teams.

Effective Communication Systems: Implementing effective communication systems, such as shared electronic health records, secure messaging platforms, and standardized communication protocols, enhances interprofessional communication. Accessible and efficient communication tools enable timely information exchange among team members.

Interprofessional Collaboration Models: Developing and implementing interprofessional collaboration models or frameworks that define healthcare professionals' roles, responsibilities, and workflows promotes effective teamwork. These models facilitate coordinated patient care, interdisciplinary rounds, shared decision-making, and collaborative care planning.

Research and Evidence: Demonstrating the value and impact of integrating pharmacists into interprofessional teams through research and evidence can generate support and facilitate the adoption of collaborative practice models. Evidence-based research on improved patient outcomes and cost-effectiveness helps overcome barriers and gain organizational buy-in.

Professional Development and Continuing Education: Offering opportunities for professional development and continuing education, such as interprofessional workshops, conferences, and training programs, allows healthcare professionals, including pharmacists, to enhance their collaborative skills and stay updated on the latest practices in team-based care.

Addressing the barriers and leveraging the facilitators can contribute to the successful integration of pharmacists in interprofessional healthcare teams. Overcoming barriers requires a concerted effort from healthcare organizations, policymakers, professional associations, and individual healthcare professionals to foster a collaborative culture and implement effective teamwork strategies. By embracing interprofessional collaboration, healthcare teams can provide patient-centered, holistic care that optimizes patient outcomes.

7. Emerging Roles for Clinical Pharmacists

Dr. Varun Singh Saggu

7.1 Pharmacogeneticists

One of the emerging roles for clinical pharmacists is that of pharmacogeneticists. Pharmacogenetics studies how an individual's genetic makeup influences their response to medications. Pharmacogeneticists specialize in applying this knowledge to personalize medication therapy based on an individual's genetic profile. Here are key aspects of the role of pharmacogeneticists:

Genetic Testing and Interpretation: Pharmacogeneticists are trained in genetic testing and interpretation. They can order and interpret genetic tests that identify specific genetic variations that affect drug metabolism, drug targets, and drug response. They have expertise in understanding how genetic variations impact the pharmacokinetics and pharmacodynamics of medications.

Medication Selection and Dosing: Pharmacogeneticists utilize genetic information to guide medication selection and dosing. By considering an individual's genetic profile, they can predict how a patient is likely to respond to specific medications and determine the most appropriate dosage. This personalized approach optimizes treatment efficacy and minimizes the risk of adverse drug reactions.

Risk Assessment and Prevention of Adverse Drug Reactions: Pharmacogeneticists can identify individuals who may be at higher risk for adverse drug reactions based on their genetic profiles. By assessing an individual's genetic predisposition to specific reactions, they can take proactive measures to minimize the risk of adverse events and prevent potential harm.

Clinical Decision Support: Pharmacogeneticists provide clinical decision support to healthcare providers by interpreting genetic data and offering recommendations based on evidence-based guidelines. They assist in analyzing complex genetic information and provide guidance on medication selection, dosing adjustments, and potential drug-drug interactions.

Education and Counseling: Pharmacogeneticists play a crucial role in educating patients and healthcare providers about the role of genetics in medication response. They counsel patients, explaining how their genetic information impacts medication therapy and helping them make informed decisions about treatment options.

Research and Collaboration: Pharmacogeneticists contribute to research in pharmacogenetics, participating in studies to further understand the impact of genetic variations on medication response. They collaborate with other healthcare professionals, researchers, and pharmacogenomic experts to advance knowledge and implementation of personalized pharmacotherapy.

Integration into Interprofessional Teams: Pharmacogeneticists work collaboratively with other healthcare professionals as part of interprofessional teams. They contribute their expertise in pharmacogenetics to inform treatment decisions, provide insights into medication therapy optimization, and enhance patient care within a team-based approach.

The role of pharmacogeneticists is continuously evolving as pharmacogenetic testing becomes more accessible, and the importance of genetic information in medication management is increasingly recognized. As precision medicine and personalized pharmacotherapy continue to advance, the expertise of pharmacogeneticists will be vital in tailoring medication therapy to individual patients based on their genetic characteristics.

7.2 Pharmacovigilance Specialists

Another emerging role for clinical pharmacists is that of pharmacovigilance specialists. Pharmacovigilance involves the monitoring, detection, assessment, and prevention of adverse effects or any other drug-related problems. Pharmacovigilance specialists ensure the safe and effective use of medications by actively monitoring and reporting adverse drug reactions (ADRs) and other medication-related issues. Here are critical aspects critical the role of pharmacovigilance specialists:

ADR Monitoring and Reporting: Pharmacovigilance specialists monitor and report ADRs and medication errors. They actively collect information on suspected ADRs from various sources, including healthcare professionals, patients, literature, and regulatory databases. They assess the severity and causality of reported events and report them to regulatory authorities to contribute to drug safety monitoring.

Risk Assessment and Signal Detection: Pharmacovigilance specialists analyze data from various sources to identify potential safety signals, trends, or emerging medication risks. They use data mining techniques and signal detection tools to identify patterns and signals that may signse previously unrecognized ADRs or safety concerns.

Safety Communication and Education: Pharmacovigilance specialists are crucial in safety communication and education. They inform healthcare professionals, patients, and other stakeholders about newly identified safety concerns, warnings, precautions, and regulatory updates. They contribute to developing educational materials and participate in training programs to enhance medication safety awareness and practices.

Pharmacovigilance Systems Development: Pharmacovigilance specialists contribute to developing and enhancing pharmacovigilance systems within healthcare organizations. They establish processes for collecting, evaluating, and reporting ADRs, ensuring compliance with regulatory requirements. They collaborate with IT professionals to develop and optimize electronic systems for efficient and streamlined pharmacovigilance activities.

Adverse Event Management: Pharmacovigilance specialists assist in managing adverse events related to medications. They collaborate with healthcare professionals to identify and manage ADRs, including dose adjustments, discontinuations, or changes in medication therapy. They provide guidance on managing medication-related problems and contribute to developing strategies to minimize harm and improve patient outcomes.

Pharmacovigilance Research: Pharmacovigilance specialists may engage in research activities related to drug safety and medication use. They contribute to post-marketing surveillance studies, observational studies, and pharmacoepidemiological research to enhance the understanding of medication safety profiles, risk factors, and mitigation strategies.

Collaboration with Regulatory Authorities and Industry: Pharmacovigilance specialists collaborate with regulatory authorities, such as the FDA, EMA, or national regulatory bodies, to ensure timely and accurate reporting of ADRs. They may also work with pharmaceutical companies and industry stakeholders to promote drug safety, provide input on risk management plans, and contribute to post-marketing surveillance activities.

The role of pharmacovigilance specialists is critical for monitoring medication safety, detecting and assessing ADRs, and contributing to the overall improvement of patient care. As the importance of pharmacovigilance in ensuring medication safety continues to grow, pharmacovigilance specialists will play a crucial role in identifying and mitigating medication-related risks, ultimately contributing to better patient outcomes and medication safety practices.

7.3 Clinical Pharmacy Consultants

Clinical pharmacy consultants are emerging roles for clinical pharmacists that involve providing specialized expertise and consultation services in various healthcare settings. These consultants offer comprehensive medication management services, clinical guidance, and evidence-based recommendations to optimize patient care. Here are critical aspects of the role of clinical pharmacy consultants:

Medication Therapy Optimization: Clinical pharmacy consultants focus on optimizing patient medication therapy. They conduct comprehensive medication reviews, assess medication regimens for appropriateness, identify drug-related problems, and make evidence-based recommendations for therapy optimization. Their expertise helps patients receive the most effective and safe medication treatment plans.

Medication Safety and Adverse Event Prevention: Clinical pharmacy consultants are crucial in medication safety and preventing adverse events. They identify and minimize medication errors, evaluate potential drug interactions, assess medication-related risks, and develop strategies to avoid adverse drug reactions. By proactively addressing medication safety concerns, they contribute to improved patient outcomes and reduced harm.

Guiding Clinical Decision-Making: Clinical pharmacy consultants provide clinical guidance and support to healthcare professionals in making informed decisions regarding medication therapy. They review patient cases, offer expertise in drug selection, dosing, and monitoring, and provide evidence-based recommendations. Their input helps healthcare teams optimize treatment plans and improve patient care.

Collaborative Care Planning: Clinical pharmacy consultants actively participate in collaborative care planning within interprofessional teams. They contribute their medication-related expertise, provide insights into drug therapy considerations, and collaborate with other healthcare professionals to develop individualized care plans. Their involvement ensures that medication management is integrated into the overall treatment approach.

Quality Improvement and Performance Measures: Clinical pharmacy consultants contribute to quality improvement initiatives by implementing and monitoring performance measures related to medication management. They evaluate medication-related outcomes, identify opportunities for improvement, and develop strategies to enhance the quality and safety of medication use.

Education and Training: Clinical pharmacy consultants play a role in educating healthcare professionals, patients, and other stakeholders about medication-related topics. They provide educational sessions, develop educational materials, and offer training programs to enhance medication knowledge and promote best practices in medication management.

Research and Evidence-Based Practice: Clinical pharmacy consultants engage in research activities and contribute to advancing evidence-based practice in pharmacy and healthcare. They participate in research projects, conduct literature reviews, and stay updated on the latest evidence to ensure their recommendations are based on the best available evidence.

Specialty-Specific Consultation: Clinical pharmacy consultants may specialize in specific areas of healthcare, such as infectious diseases, critical care, oncology, or pediatrics. Their specialized knowledge and experience allow them to provide expert consultation and guidance in their respective areas of expertise.

Clinical pharmacy consultants bring specialized medication expertise to healthcare teams, ensuring comprehensive and optimized medication management. Their involvement helps improve patient outcomes, enhance medication safety, promote evidence-based practice, and contribute to quality improvement initiatives within healthcare settings.

7.3 Clinical Pharmacy Consultants

Clinical pharmacy consultants are emerging roles for clinical pharmacists that involve providing specialized expertise and consultation services in various healthcare settings. These consultants offer comprehensive medication management services, clinical guidance, and evidence-based recommendations to optimize patient care. Here are critical aspects of the role of clinical pharmacy consultants:

Medication Therapy Optimization: Clinical pharmacy consultants focus on optimizing patient medication therapy. They conduct comprehensive medication reviews, assess medication regimens for appropriateness, identify drug-related problems, and make evidence-based recommendations for therapy optimization. Their expertise helps patients receive the most effective and safe medication treatment plans.

Medication Safety and Adverse Event Prevention: Clinical pharmacy consultants are crucial in medication safety and preventing adverse events. They identify and minimize medication errors, evaluate potential drug interactions, assess medication-related risks, and develop strategies to prevent avoid drug reactions. By proactively addressing medication safety concerns, they contribute to improved patient outcomes and reduced harm.

Guiding Clinical Decision-Making: Clinical pharmacy consultants provide clinical guidance and support to healthcare professionals in making informed decisions regarding medication therapy. They review patient cases, offer expertise in drug selection, dosing, and monitoring, and provide evidence-based recommendations. Their input helps healthcare teams optimize treatment plans and improve patient care.

Collaborative Care Planning: Clinical pharmacy consultants actively participate in collaborative care planning within interprofessional teams. They contribute their medication-related expertise, provide insights into drug therapy considerations, and collaborate with other healthcare professionals to develop individualized care plans. Their involvement ensures that medication management is integrated into the overall treatment approach.

Quality Improvement and Performance Measures: Clinical pharmacy consultants contribute to quality improvement initiatives by implementing and monitoring performance measures related to medication management. They evaluate medication-related outcomes, identify opportunities for improvement, and develop strategies to enhance the quality and safety of medication use.

Education and Training: Clinical pharmacy consultants play a role in educating healthcare professionals, patients, and other stakeholders about medication-related topics. They provide educational sessions, develop educational materials, and offer training programs to enhance medication knowledge and promote best practices in medication management.

Research and Evidence-Based Practice: Clinical pharmacy consultants engage in research activities and contribute to advancing evidence-based practice in pharmacy and healthcare. They participate in research projects, conduct literature reviews, and stay updated on the latest evidence to ensure their recommendations are based on the best available evidence.

Specialty-Specific Consultation: Clinical pharmacy consultants may specialize in specific areas of healthcare, such as infectious diseases, critical care, oncology, or pediatrics. Their specialized knowledge and experience allow them to provide expert consultation and guidance in their respective areas of expertise.

Clinical pharmacy consultants bring specialized medication expertise to healthcare teams, ensuring comprehensive and optimized medication management. Their involvement helps improve patient outcomes, enhance medication safety, promote evidence-based practice, and contribute to quality improvement initiatives within healthcare settings.

7.4 Transitions of Care Pharmacists

Transitions of care pharmacists are emerging roles for clinical pharmacists that focus on ensuring safe and seamless transitions of patients between different healthcare settings, such as hospitals, rehabilitation facilities, long-term care facilities, and home care. These pharmacists are crucial in coordinating medication management during care transitions and optimizing medication therapy for patients. Here are key aspects role of changes of care pharmacists:

Medication Reconciliation: Transitions of care pharmacists are responsible for conducting medication reconciliation, which involves comparing patients' medication lists as they move between different healthcare settings. They identify discrepancies, resolve medication-related issues, and ensure accurate and up-to-date medication information is available to healthcare providers and patients.

Continuity of Medication Therapy: Transitions of care pharmacists ensure continuity of medication therapy during care transitions. They collaborate with healthcare professionals involved in the patient's care to provide accurate medication information, including dosages, frequency, and administration instructions. They facilitate the seamless transfer of medication orders and assist in the procurement and delivery of medications.

Patient Education and Medication Counseling: Transitions of care pharmacists educate patients and caregivers about their medications during care transitions. They provide medication counseling, including information on medication indications, potential side effects, proper administration, and adherence strategies. They also address any concerns or questions related to medication therapy to promote patient understanding and engagement.

Medication Optimization and Safety: Transitions of care pharmacists optimize medication therapy during transitions to ensure safe and effective use of medications. They review medication regimens, assess potential drug interactions or duplications, and make recommendations for therapy adjustments. They also identify and address medication-related risks, such as adverse drug reactions or drug allergies, to enhance patient safety.

Care Coordination and Communication: Transitions of care pharmacists collaborate with healthcare professionals across different settings to facilitate care coordination and effective communication. They actively communicate medication-related information, including changes in therapy, dose adjustments, or new medications, to ensure continuity of care. They also provide timely and accurate medication-related documentation to support interdisciplinary communication.

Medication Adherence Support: Transitions of care pharmacists assist patients in maintaining medication adherence during care transitions. They provide strategies and resources to promote adherence, such as medication organizers, reminder systems, and refill management. They also identify and address barriers to adherence, such as cost or access issues, and collaborate with healthcare providers to find appropriate solutions.

Transitions Planning and Follow-up: Transitions of care pharmacists contribute to transitions planning and follow-up care. They participate in discharge planning, medication counseling sessions, and medication-related care plans. They ensure that patients have appropriate medications and supplies upon discharge and collaborate with community pharmacists and other healthcare providers to facilitate follow-up care and medication-related monitoring.

Quality Improvement Initiatives: Transitions of care pharmacists actively participate in quality improvement initiatives related to medication management during care transitions. They contribute to developing and implementing standardized processes, protocols, and performance measures to enhance the quality and safety of medication transitions. They also analyze data and outcomes to identify areas for improvement and implement evidence-based practices.

The role of transitions of care pharmacists is critical in minimizing medication-related errors, ensuring medication continuity, and optimizing patient outcomes during care transitions. By actively engaging in medication reconciliation, education, optimization, and coordination, transitions of care pharmacists enhance patient safety, improve medication adherence, and contribute to the overall quality of care during transitions between healthcare settings.

7.5 Clinical Research Pharmacists

Clinical research pharmacists are emerging roles for clinical pharmacists who specialize in conducting and managing clinical research studies. They play a crucial role in the design, implementation, and evaluation of clinical trials and other research projects related to pharmaceuticals. Here are key aspects of the role of clinical research pharmacists:

Protocol Development: Clinical research pharmacists actively contribute to the development of research protocols. They provide expertise in medication-related aspects, such as study drug selection, dosing, administration, and monitoring. They ensure that the protocols align with ethical and regulatory requirements and contribute to the scientific rigor of the study.

Investigational Drug Management: Clinical research pharmacists are responsible for the management and oversight of investigational drugs used in clinical trials. They ensure the appropriate storage, handling, dispensing, and accountability of study drugs, following good clinical practice (GCP) guidelines and regulatory requirements.

Participant Recruitment and Informed Consent: Clinical research pharmacists assist in participant recruitment efforts for clinical trials. They educate potential participants about the study, including the purpose, risks, benefits, and potential side effects of the investigational drug. They also ensure that participants provide informed consent before enrolling in the study.

Study Execution and Data Collection: Clinical research pharmacists actively participate in the execution of clinical trials. They collaborate with the research team to ensure accurate data collection, monitor participant adherence to study protocols, and manage any medication-related issues that arise during the study. They also contribute to data quality assurance and adherence to regulatory requirements.

Pharmacokinetic and Pharmacodynamic Monitoring: Clinical research pharmacists play a key role in pharmacokinetic and pharmacodynamic monitoring during clinical trials. They design and implement monitoring plans, collect and analyze pharmacokinetic data, and evaluate the relationship between drug concentrations and therapeutic response. This information contributes to the understanding of drug efficacy and safety profiles.

Adverse Event Monitoring and Reporting: Clinical research pharmacists are responsible for monitoring and reporting adverse events that occur during clinical trials. They assess the severity and causality of adverse events, ensure appropriate documentation, and report them to regulatory authorities and the research team according to regulatory requirements.

Collaborative Research Team Engagement: Clinical research pharmacists actively collaborate with other members of the research team, including principal investigators, study coordinators, and data managers. They contribute their medication expertise, provide guidance on study drug-related matters, and ensure seamless communication and coordination among team members.

Compliance with Regulatory and Ethical Requirements: Clinical research pharmacists ensure compliance with regulatory and ethical requirements throughout the research process. They stay updated on current regulations, guidelines, and ethical considerations related to clinical research and ensure adherence to these requirements in all aspects of the study.

Data Analysis and Publication: Clinical research pharmacists contribute to data analysis and interpretation of study results. They collaborate with statisticians and researchers to analyze study data, interpret findings, and contribute to the publication of study results in scientific journals or presentations at conferences.

Clinical research pharmacists play a vital role in advancing pharmaceutical knowledge and improving patient care through their involvement in clinical trials and research projects. Their expertise in medication management, pharmacokinetics, and regulatory requirements ensures the integrity, safety, and ethical conduct of clinical research studies.

8. Contemporary Issues in Clinical Pharmacy

Dr. Varun Singh Saggu

8.1 Medication Safety and Quality Assurance

Medication safety and quality assurance are significant contemporary issues in clinical pharmacy. Ensuring the safe and effective use of medications is a priority for healthcare professionals, including clinical pharmacists. Here are key aspects of medication safety and quality assurance:

Medication Errors: Medication errors can occur at any stage of the medication use process, including prescribing, dispensing, administering, and monitoring. Clinical pharmacists play a vital role in preventing and mitigating medication errors through medication reconciliation, comprehensive medication reviews, error reporting systems, and implementation of safety protocols.

Adverse Drug Events: Adverse drug events (ADEs) refer to harm caused by medication use, including adverse drug reactions, medication errors, and medication-related incidents. Clinical pharmacists contribute to ADE prevention by conducting medication assessments, monitoring drug interactions and adverse effects, and providing medication counseling to minimize the risk of ADEs.

Medication Reconciliation: Medication reconciliation is the process of comparing a patient's current medication regimen to their intended medication regimen during care transitions. Clinical pharmacists play a crucial role in medication reconciliation to identify and resolve medication discrepancies, reduce medication errors, and ensure accurate medication lists across different healthcare settings.

High-Risk Medications: Certain medications are considered high-risk due to their potential for harm or complexity. Clinical pharmacists focus on the safe use of high-risk medications by conducting risk assessments, implementing risk mitigation strategies, monitoring patients closely, and providing education to healthcare professionals and patients on their appropriate use.

Quality Assurance Programs: Clinical pharmacists contribute to quality assurance programs that aim to improve medication safety and quality of care. They participate in medication safety committees, engage in medication utilization evaluations, develop medication-related policies and guidelines, and collaborate with interdisciplinary teams to implement best practices and enhance patient safety.

Technology and Automation: Technology and automation solutions, such as electronic prescribing systems, barcode scanning, and automated dispensing systems, play a significant role in medication safety and quality assurance. Clinical pharmacists are involved in the implementation, optimization, and oversight of these technologies to minimize medication errors and improve the accuracy of medication-related processes.

Adherence and Patient Education: Medication adherence is critical for achieving optimal therapeutic outcomes. Clinical pharmacists focus on promoting medication adherence by providing patient education, counseling, and adherence support strategies. They collaborate with healthcare teams to address barriers to adherence and enhance patient understanding and self-management of medications.

Continuous Quality Improvement: Clinical pharmacists actively participate in continuous quality improvement initiatives to enhance medication safety and quality of care. They analyze medication-related data, participate in root cause analyses of medication errors or ADEs, implement evidence-based practices, and contribute to performance improvement measures to drive positive changes in medication safety.

Regulatory and Accreditation Standards: Clinical pharmacists ensure compliance with regulatory and accreditation standards related to medication safety and quality assurance. They stay updated on medication-related regulations, guidelines, and bars, implement necessary policies and procedures, and contribute to medication-related audits and inspections.

Medication safety and quality assurance remain ongoing concerns in clinical pharmacy. Clinical pharmacists, through their expertise and collaboration with other healthcare professionals, strive to optimize medication use, prevent medication errors, and improve patient outcomes by promoting safe and effective medication practices.

8.2 Drug Pricing and Affordability

Drug pricing and affordability is a significant contemporary issue in clinical pharmacy. The cost of medications has been rising, making them increasingly unaffordable for many patients. Here are key aspects of drug pricing and affordability:

Rising Drug Costs: The cost of prescription drugs has been increasing at a significant rate, often outpacing inflation and putting a financial burden on patients and healthcare systems. The high cost of medications can limit access to essential treatments and potentially compromise patient outcomes.

Access to Essential Medications: The high cost of certain medications can create barriers to access, particularly for individuals without adequate insurance coverage or those with limited financial resources. This issue affects patients' ability to obtain necessary medications and can lead to medication non-adherence or the use of alternative, potentially fewer effective treatments.

Health Disparities: High drug costs contribute to health disparities, as patients from low-income backgrounds or underserved populations may face greater challenges in accessing and affording medications. This can exacerbate existing health inequities and lead to unequal healthcare outcomes.

Medication Adherence: Affordability plays a crucial role in medication adherence. Patients who cannot afford their medications may skip doses, split pills, or delay refills, compromising treatment efficacy and patient safety. Clinical pharmacists work with patients to address affordability issues and explore options such as assistance programs, generic alternatives, or therapeutic alternatives.

Value-Based Pricing: Value-based pricing models aim to align drug prices with the clinical and economic value they provide. Clinical pharmacists can contribute to assessing the value of medications by evaluating clinical outcomes, cost-effectiveness, and patient-centered outcomes. This information can inform discussions around drug pricing and support informed decision-making.

Formulary Management: Clinical pharmacists play a role in formulary management within healthcare organizations. They contribute to selecting medications for formularies based on efficacy, safety, and cost considerations. Clinical pharmacists may engage in cost-effectiveness evaluations and work with other stakeholders to ensure the inclusion of affordable medications in formularies.

Medication Assistance Programs: Clinical pharmacists can help patients navigate medication assistance programs and identify options for reducing out-of-pocket costs. They provide guidance on patient assistance programs, manufacturer discounts, and other financial assistance resources to help patients access affordable medications.

Advocacy and Policy Engagement: Clinical pharmacists can advocate for policy changes and reforms aimed at addressing drug pricing and affordability. They can engage in professional organizations, work with policymakers, and contribute to discussions on healthcare reform to advocate for measures that promote access to affordable medications.

Education and Patient Empowerment: Clinical pharmacists play a role in educating patients about the cost of medications and available options for reducing costs. They can provide information on generic equivalents, therapeutic alternatives, and strategies for improving medication affordability. Patient education empowers patients to make informed decisions about their medications and explore cost-saving opportunities.

Addressing drug pricing and affordability requires a multifaceted approach involving collaboration among healthcare professionals, policymakers, pharmaceutical companies, and other stakeholders. Clinical pharmacists have an essential role in advocating for affordable medications, exploring cost-saving strategies, and helping patients navigate the complex landscape of medication costs to ensure access to necessary treatments and improve patient outcomes.

8.3 Pharmaceutical Industry Influence

Pharmaceutical industry influence is a significant contemporary issue in clinical pharmacy. The pharmaceutical industry's influence can impact various aspects of healthcare, including research, drug development, prescribing practices, and healthcare policies. Here are key aspects of pharmaceutical industry's influence:

Research and Clinical Trials: The pharmaceutical industry plays a significant role in funding and conducting clinical trials and research studies. While industry-sponsored research contributes to scientific knowledge and the development of new therapies, there is a concern that industry-funded studies may be biased towards favorable outcomes or may selectively publish results, potentially influencing clinical practice.

Drug Promotion and Marketing: Pharmaceutical companies heavily market their products to healthcare professionals, including clinical pharmacists. Direct-to-physician marketing sponsored educational events and promotional materials may influence prescribing behaviors and increase the utilization of specific medications, even if alternative, equally effective, and more affordable options are available.

Financial Relationships: Pharmaceutical companies often establish financial relationships with healthcare professionals, including clinical pharmacists, through consulting fees, research grants, speaking engagements, and sponsorship of educational events. These financial relationships can raise concerns about potential conflicts of interest and their impact on professional judgment and prescribing practices.

Formulary Decision-Making: Pharmaceutical industry influence extends to formulary decision-making within healthcare organizations. Manufacturers may exert influence through pricing negotiations, rebates, and other financial incentives to ensure favorable product formulary placement. This can impact medication availability, affordability, and utilization within healthcare systems.

Access to Clinical Trial Data: There has been growing concern about the need for more transparency and limited access to complete clinical trial data. Pharmaceutical companies may selectively release trial data, potentially obscuring adverse or unfavorable outcomes. Access to complete trial data is crucial for evidence-based decision-making and unbiased evaluation of drug efficacy and safety.

Direct-to-Consumer Advertising: Pharmaceutical companies can influence patients' perceptions and demands for specific medications.

This may contribute to increased patient requests for advertised medications, potentially influencidrugsing decisions by healthcare professionals, including clinical pharmacists.

Drug Pricing and Affordability: The pharmaceutical industry's pricing practices and strategies can significantly impact the affordability of medications. High drug prices, price hikes, and pricing disparities among different regions or countries can limit patient access to necessary treatments and pose financial burdens on healthcare systems.

Influence on Healthcare Policies: The pharmaceutical industry influences healthcare policies through lobbying efforts, advocacy campaigns, and involvement in policy development processes. This influence can shape healthcare legislation, regulations, and procedures related to drug pricing, intellectual property rights, generic competition, and reimbursement systems.

Conflict of Interest Disclosure and Management: Recognizing and managing conflicts of interest is essential in maintaining the integrity and objectivity of clinical pharmacy practice. Clinical pharmacists should disclose potential conflicts of interest and ensure transparent patient care, research, and formulary management decision-making processes.

Addressing the pharmaceutical industry's influence requires transparency, ethics, and robust policies. Clinical pharmacists and healthcare organizations should promote evidence-based decision-making, ensure transparency in financial relationships, implement rigorous conflict-of-interest management strategies, and advocate for policies that prioritizingent welfare, affordability, and unbiased prescribing practices.

8.4 Medication Adherence Challenges

Medication adherence challenges are significant contemporary issues in clinical pharmacy. Medication adherence refers to the extent to which patients take medications as prescribed by their healthcare providers. Non-adherence can have detrimental effects on treatment outcomes and patient health. Here are keycriticalpects of medication adherence challenges:

Complex Medication Regimens: Many patients are prescribed complex medication regimens that involve multiple medications, various dosing schedules, and specific instructions. Managing and adhering to such regimens can be challenging for patients, leading to confusion, errors, and non-adherence.

Lack of Patient Understanding: Limited health literacy, language barriers, and adequate patient education can contribute to better medication understanding and non-adherence. Patients may have difficulty comprehending medication labels, instructions, and the importance of medication adherence, resulting in suboptimal treatment outcomes.

Side Effects and Perceived Benefits: Medication side effects can deter patients from adhering to their prescribed regimen. If patients experience unpleasant side effects or do not perceive immediate benefits from their medications, they may be less motivated to continue taking them as prescribed, leading to non-adherence.

Affordability and Access: The cost of medications and lack of insurance coverage can pose significant barriers to medication adherence. Patients may skip doses or discontinue medications to reduce costs. Limited access to pharmacies or healthcare facilities can also hinder patients' ability to obtain their medications consistently.

Forgetfulness and Lack of Reminder Systems: Forgetfulness is a common reason for medication non-adherence. Patients may simply forget to take their medications as scheduled. Lack of reminder systems, such as pill organizers, medication alarms, or mobile apps, can contribute to forgetfulness and non-adherence.

Mental Health and Cognitive Factors: Mental health conditions, such as depression, anxiety, or cognitive impairment, can impact medication adherence. Patients experiencing these conditions may have difficulty remembering to take their medications or lack the motivation to adhere to their prescribed regimen.

Social and Cultural Factors: Social and cultural factors can influence medication adherence. Patient beliefs, attitudes, cultural norms, and social support networks may impact adherence behaviors. The stigma associated with certain conditions or medications may also affect patients' willingness to adhere to their prescribed regimen.

Polypharmacy and Medication Interactions: Patients taking multiple medications face a higher risk of non-adherence. Complex medication regimens, potential medication interactions, and managing multiple prescription refills can lead to confusion and non-adherence.

Healthcare System Factors: Healthcare system factors, such as limited appointment time, lack of continuity of care, and fragmented healthcare delivery, can contribute to medication adherence challenges. Inadequate communication between healthcare providers and patients, insufficient medication counseling, and insufficient follow-up can hinder adherence.

Addressing medication adherence challenges requires a multi-faceted approach involving healthcare professionals, patients, and healthcare systems. Clinical pharmacists can play a pivotal role in addressing adherence challenges by providing patient education, simplifying medication regimens, implementing reminder systems, assessing affordability and access issues, and collaborating with other healthcare providers to enhance patient understanding and adherence. Patient-centered strategies, tailored interventions, and collaborative efforts are necessary to improve medication adherence and optimize treatment outcomes.

8.5 Global Health and Access to Medicines

Global health and access to medicines are pressing contemporary issues in clinical pharmacy. Access to affordable and essential medications is crucial for promoting equitable healthcare worldwide. Here are critical aspects of global health and access to medicines:

Health Inequities: Global health disparities and inequities affect access to medicines. Low- and middle-income countries often face challenges in accessing affordable and essential medications due to limited healthcare infrastructure, inadequate funding, and regulatory barriers. Addressing health inequities is critical for ensuring access to medicines for all individuals, regardless of their geographic location or socioeconomic status.

High Drug Prices: High drug prices can significantly limit medication access, particularly in low- and middle-income countries. Patents, intellectual property rights, and market exclusivity can contribute to monopolies and prevent generic competition, resulting in inflated prices. Reducing drug prices and ensuring fair pricing strategies are vital for improving access to affordable medications globally.

Essential Medicines: The World Health Organization (WHO) defines crucial medicines as medications that are necessary for addressing priority health needs in a healthcare system. However, access to essential medicines remains a challenge in many parts of the world. Clinical pharmacists can advocate for the availability and affordability of essential medicines to ensure equitable access to these vital treatments.

Supply Chain and Distribution Challenges: Inadequate supply chain management and distribution systems can hinder access to medicines in remote or underserved areas. Clinical pharmacists can play a role in optimizing supply chain processes and collaborating with other stakeholders to ensure the reliable and efficient delivery of medications to all communities, including those in resource-limited settings.

Rational Use of Medicines: The rational use of medicines involves prescribing and using medications appropriately, based on scientific evidence and patient needs. Promoting rational use can improve access to effective treatments while reducing unnecessary costs and the risk of antimicrobial resistance. Clinical pharmacists contribute to rational use through medication reviews, providing evidence-based recommendations, and educating healthcare professionals and patients on appropriate medication use.

Global Health Partnerships: Collaboration among countries, international organizations, pharmaceutical companies, and healthcare professionals is essential for addressing global health challenges and improving access to medicines. Clinical pharmacists can actively participate in global health partnerships, knowledge sharing, capacity building, and initiatives aimed at enhancing access to affordable medications worldwide.

Generic Medications: Generic medications offer cost-effective alternatives to brand-name drugs. Promoting the use of quality-assured generic medications can significantly improve access to essential treatments, particularly in resource-limited settings. Clinical pharmacists play a role in educating healthcare professionals and patients about the safety, efficacy, and affordability of generic medications.

Sustainable Development Goals: The United Nations Sustainable Development Goals (SDGs) include specific targets related to health, access to medicines, and universal health coverage. Clinical pharmacists can contribute to achieving these goals by advocating for policies and practices that prioritize access to affordable medicines, promoting evidence-based and cost-effective prescribing, and supporting initiatives that enhance the healthcare system's capacity to provide equitable access to medicines.

Addressing global health and access to medicines requires a comprehensive and collaborative approach involving governments, policymakers, healthcare professionals, pharmaceutical companies, and international organizations. Clinical pharmacists, through their expertise in medication management, evidence-based practice, and advocacy, can play a vital role in promoting equitable access to affordable medicines and contributing to global health initiatives.

9. Future Perspectives in Clinical Pharmacy

Dr. Varun Singh Saggu

9.1 Artificial Intelligence and Machine Learning

Artificial intelligence (AI) and machine learning (ML) hold immense potential for the future of clinical pharmacy. These technologies can revolutionize various aspects of medication management, patient care, and decision-making processes. Here are key future perspectives of AI and ML in clinical pharmacy:

Medication Management and Optimization: AI and ML algorithms can assist in medication management by analyzing patient data, including medical history, genetic information, and clinical parameters, to optimize medication selection, dosing, and monitoring. These technologies can identify patterns, predict treatment outcomes, and provide personalized recommendations for medication therapy.

Clinical Decision Support Systems: AI and ML can enhance clinical decision support systems by providing real-time, evidence-based recommendations to healthcare professionals. These technologies can analyze patient data, consider relevant guidelines and literature, and generate alerts or suggestions for drug interactions, adverse drug reactions, dosing adjustments, and medication adherence.

Pharmacogenomics and Personalized Medicine: AI and ML algorithms can analyze genomic data and identify genetic markers influencing drug response. By integrating pharmacogenomic information with patient-specific clinical data, these technologies can enable personalized medicine approaches, optimizing medication selection and dosing based on an individual's genetic profile.

Drug Discovery and Development: AI and ML can expedite the drug discovery and development process by analyzing vast amounts of biomedical data, identifying potential drug targets, and predicting the efficacy and safety of drug candidates. These technologies can enhance the efficiency of preclinical and clinical trials, leading to faster and more accurate drug development.

Adverse Event Detection and Pharmacovigilance: AI and ML can improve negative event detection and pharmacovigilance by analyzing real-world data, including electronic health records, social media posts, and drug safety databases. These technologies can identify signals of potential adverse events, assess causality, and contribute to early detection and mitigation of medication-related risks.

Predictive Analytics and Population Health Management: AI and ML algorithms can analyze population-level health data to predict disease trends, medication utilization patterns, and medication-related outcomes. This information can assist in population health management, resource allocation, and targeted interventions to improve patient outcomes and optimize healthcare delivery.

Patient Engagement and Adherence: AI-powered chatbots, mobile applications, and virtual assistants can support patient engagement and medication adherence. These technologies can provide personalized medication reminders, educational materials, and real-time support, empowering patients to participate in their medication management and make informed decisions actively.

Data Privacy and Ethical Considerations: Integrating AI and ML in clinical pharmacy raises essential considerations regarding data privacy, security, and ethical use of patient information. Safeguarding patient data, ensuring transparency in algorithmic decision-making, and maintaining patient trust are crucial aspects that need to be addressed in the future deployment of AI and ML technologies.

The future of clinical pharmacy is closely intertwined with the advancements in AI and ML. Integrating these technologies into practice can enhance medication management, improve patient outcomes, enable personalized medicine approaches, and optimize healthcare delivery. However, it is vital to ensure ethical use, address potential biases, and maintain a patient-centered approach in implementing AI and ML in clinical pharmacy.

9.2 Virtual Reality and Augmented Reality

Virtual reality (VR) and augmented reality (AR) technologies offer exciting future perspectives in clinical pharmacy. These immersive technologies can potentially enhance medication education, training, and patient care. Here are critical future views of VR and AR in clinical pharmacy:

Medication Education and Training: VR and AR can provide immersive and interactive medication education and training platforms. In a realistic virtual environment, students and healthcare professionals can simulate medication administration, dosage calculations, and medication counseling scenarios. This technology can enhance learning outcomes, promote skill development, and improve medication-related competencies.

Medication Safety and Error Prevention: VR and AR can create virtual environments where healthcare professionals can practice medication safety protocols and error prevention strategies. These simulations can help identify potential risks, improve decision-making skills, and enhance situational awareness to prevent medication errors in real-world settings.

Patient Counseling and Adherence Support: VR and AR can facilitate patient counseling and medication adherence support. By using virtual simulations, healthcare professionals can visually demonstrate medication administration techniques, provide medication counseling, and address patient concerns in an engaging and immersive manner. This technology can improve patient understanding, adherence, and self-management of medications.

Telepharmacy and Remote Consultations: VR and AR technologies can enhance telepharmacy services and remote consultations. Healthcare professionals can use virtual platforms to interact with patients in real-time, visually assess medication adherence, and provide medication counseling remotely. This technology can improve access to clinical pharmacy services, especially in underserved or remote areas.

Medication Reconciliation and Decision Support: VR and AR can support medication reconciliation processes and clinical decision-making. Through immersive interfaces, healthcare professionals can review and compare medication lists, identify discrepancies, and make informed decisions regarding medication regimens. This technology can improve medication reconciliation practices' accuracy, efficiency, and patient safety.

Enhanced Patient Engagement and Empowerment: VR and AR can improve patient engagement and empowerment in medication management. Patients can use AR-enabled mobile applications or wearable devices to access personalized medication information, receive medication reminders, and access educational materials. This technology can promote patient involvement in their healthcare, improve medication adherence, and empower patients to make informed decisions.

Medication Visualization and Therapy Monitoring: VR and AR can visualize the effects of medications on the body and monitor therapy progress. Healthcare professionals can use immersive technology to show patients how drugs interact with specific organs or systems, enhancing patient understanding of treatment mechanisms. These technologies can also facilitate real-time monitoring of medication responses, such as changes in vital signs or biomarkers.

Collaboration and Interprofessional Communication: VR and AR can facilitate cooperation and communication among healthcare professionals. By creating virtual environments, healthcare teams can remotely collaborate on medication-related cases, discuss treatment plans, and share expertise across different locations. This technology can improve interprofessional collaboration and enhance patient care outcomes.

While VR and AR technologies offer promising future perspectives in clinical pharmacy, it is essential to address challenges such as cost, accessibility, and data privacy. Additionally, these technologies must be validated and standardized to ensure their effectiveness, reliability, and integration into clinical pharmacy practice.

9.3 Nanotechnology in Drug Delivery

Nanotechnology holds great promise for the future of drug delivery in clinical pharmacy. Nanoparticles and nanoscale materials offer unique properties that enhance drug solubility, stability, targeted delivery, and controlled release. Here are key future perspectives of nanotechnology in drug delivery:

Enhanced Drug Solubility and Bioavailability: Nanotechnology can address the solubility challenges of poorly water-soluble drugs. Nanoparticles can encapsulate hydrophobic drugs, improving their solubility and bioavailability. This technology enables the development of more effective oral, injectable, and topical formulations for improved drug delivery.

Targeted Drug Delivery: Nanoparticles can be engineered to deliver drugs to specific target sites, such as tumors or inflamed tissues.

Functionalized nanoparticles can recognize and bind to specific receptors or markers, allowing targeted drug delivery and reducing off-target effects. This technology enhances therapeutic efficacy while minimizing side effects.

Controlled and Sustained Drug Release: Nanotechnology enables precise control over drug release kinetics. Nanoparticles can be designed to release drugs sustainably, providing prolonged therapeutic effects and reducing the frequency of dosing. This controlled release can improve patient convenience, compliance, and therapeutic outcomes.

Theranostics and Imaging: Nanoparticles can serve as theranostic agents by combining therapeutic and diagnostic functions. They can carry drugs while also acting as contrast agents for imaging techniques, such as magnetic resonance imaging (MRI) or computed tomography (CT). This integrated approach enables simultaneous diagnosis and treatment monitoring.

Personalized Medicine: Nanotechnology offers opportunities for personalized medicine approaches. Nanoparticles can be tailored to individual patient needs, considering factors such as disease characteristics, genetic variations, and drug responses. This customization enables more precise drug delivery and personalized treatment strategies.

Combination Therapy: Nanoparticles can deliver multiple drugs simultaneously, enabling combination therapy approaches. This approach can improve therapeutic outcomes by targeting multiple disease pathways or synergistic drug effects. Nanotechnology enables the co-encapsulation or sequential release of different drugs, enhancing treatment efficacy.

Vaccine Delivery: Nanoparticles can enhance vaccine delivery and immunization strategies. They can improve antigen stability, facilitate targeted antigen delivery to immune cells, and enhance immune responses. This technology can potentially improve vaccine effectiveness, reduce dosage requirements, and enable novel vaccination approaches.

Regenerative Medicine: Nanotechnology can contribute to the field of regenerative medicine. Nanomaterials can act as scaffolds for tissue engineering, providing a supportive matrix for cell growth and regeneration. Nanoparticles can deliver growth factors, stem cells, or genetic material to facilitate tissue repair and regeneration.

Safety and Toxicity Considerations: Nanotechnology offers exciting opportunities, addressing safety and toxicity concerns is crucial. The potential impact of nanoparticles on biological systems, long-term effects, and potential accumulation in organs should be thoroughly evaluated to ensure patient safety.

The future integration of nanotechnology in drug delivery has the potential to revolutionize clinical pharmacy. It can enhance drug efficacy, improve patient outcomes, and enable personalized medicine approaches. Continued research, collaboration, and regulatory considerations are necessary to harness the full potential of nanotechnology in clinical practice.

9.4 Blockchain Technology in Pharmacy

Blockchain technology has the potential to revolutionize various aspects of pharmacy practice, including medication management, supply chain transparency, and patient data security. Here are key future perspectives of blockchain technology in clinical pharmacy:

Medication Traceability and Supply Chain Transparency: Blockchain can provide a transparent and immutable record of the entire medication supply chain, from manufacturing to dispensing.

This technology can enhance drug traceability, reducing the risk of counterfeit medications and ensuring the authenticity and quality of pharmaceutical products.

Drug Authentication and Anti-Counterfeiting: Blockchain-based systems can enable real-time verification of medication authenticity and provenance. Patients, healthcare providers, and pharmacists can access secure and decentralized databases to verify the legitimacy of medications, mitigating the risks associated with counterfeit drugs.

Electronic Health Records (EHR) Security and Interoperability: Blockchain can enhance the security and interoperability of electronic health records. It enables secure sharing and exchange of patient health data between healthcare providers while ensuring data integrity, privacy, and consent management. Blockchain-based EHR systems can reduce data breaches, improve data accessibility, and empower patients to have more control over their health information.

Medication Adherence and Smart Contracts: Blockchain-based smart contracts can facilitate medication adherence by automating medication reminders, refill notifications, and adherence monitoring. These contracts can be programmed to trigger alerts and incentives for patients who adhere to their prescribed medication regimens, enhancing patient engagement and adherence.

Clinical Trials and Research Data Management: Blockchain can improve the integrity and transparency of clinical trial data. By using blockchain technology, researchers can securely store and share trial data, ensuring transparency, traceability, and immutability. This technology can enhance data integrity, streamline research collaboration, and enable more efficient clinical trial processes.

Drug Recall Management: Blockchain-based systems can facilitate more efficient and transparent drug recall management. The decentralized nature of blockchain allows for real-time tracking of affected medications, ensuring prompt and targeted recall processes. This technology can minimize the impact of drug recalls on patient safety and streamline recall communication between manufacturers, regulators, and healthcare providers.

Drug Pricing Transparency: Blockchain technology has the potential to increase pricing transparency in the pharmaceutical industry. By recording and tracking the entire supply chain, including pricing information, blockchain can enhance visibility into the costs associated with drug development, manufacturing, and distribution. This transparency can potentially facilitate fairer pricing practices and improve access to affordable medications.

Prescription Drug Abuse and Controlled Substance Monitoring: Blockchain can contribute to the monitoring and prevention of prescription drug abuse. By creating an immutable record of controlled substance prescriptions and tracking their dispensing, blockchain technology can facilitate the detection of inappropriate or excessive medication use, support regulatory compliance, and mitigate the risks associated with prescription drug abuse.

While blockchain technology offers promising future perspectives in clinical pharmacy, challenges such as scalability, interoperability, and regulatory considerations need to be addressed. Collaboration among stakeholders, research, and pilot implementations are necessary to harness the full potential of blockchain technology in pharmacy practice and ensure its secure and effective integration.

9.5 Emerging Therapeutic Approaches

Emerging therapeutic approaches hold great promise for the future of clinical pharmacy, offering innovative ways to treat diseases and improve patient outcomes. Here are key future perspectives of emerging therapeutic approaches in clinical pharmacy:

Gene Therapy: Gene therapy involves the delivery of genetic material to treat or prevent diseases caused by congenital abnormalities. It holds the potential for treating genetic disorders, certain types of cancer, and other conditions. Clinical pharmacists can play a role in gene therapy by ensuring appropriate medication management, monitoring treatment responses, and providing patient education these therapies' benefits and potential risks pies.

Immunotherapy: Immunotherapy harnesses the power of the immune system to combat diseases, including cancer. It includes approaches such as immune checkpoint inhibitors, CAR-T cell therapy, and therapeutic vaccines. Clinical pharmacists can contribute to immunotherapy by managing immunosuppressive medications, monitoring for immune-related adverse events, and educating patients on treatment expectations and side effects.

Precision Medicine: Precision medicine focuses on individualized treatment approaches based on a patient's unique characteristics, including genetic makeup, biomarker profiles, and clinical data. Clinical pharmacists play a vital role in precision medicine by interpreting genetic test results, optimizing medication therapy based on genomic information, and collaborating with healthcare teams to develop personalized treatment plans.

Nanomedicine: Nanomedicine involves using nanoscale materials and nanoparticles for targeted drug delivery, imaging, and diagnostics. Clinical pharmacists can contribute to nanomedicine by understanding nanotechnology principles, monitoring treatment responses, and ensuring nanomedicines' safe and effective use.

Stem Cell Therapy: Stem cell therapy utilizes the regenerative properties of stem cells to repair damaged tissues and treat various diseases. It holds promise for conditions such as neurodegenerative disorders, cardiovascular diseases, and certain types of cancer. Clinical pharmacists can support stem cell therapy by managing medications during transplantation, monitoring for adverse events, and providing medication counseling to patients.

RNA-based Therapies: RNA-based therapies, such as messenger RNA (mRNA) vaccines and RNA interference (RNAi) therapies, offer innovative approaches to target specific genes and modulate protein expression. Clinical pharmacists can contribute to RNA-based therapies by monitoring treatment responses, managing associated medications, and educating patients about the benefits and potential side effects of these therapies.

Digital Therapeutics: Digital therapeutics are software-based interventions that aim to prevent, manage, or treat medical conditions. They often involve smartphone applications, wearables, and online platforms to deliver personalized interventions and support patient self-management. Clinical pharmacists can integrate digital therapeutics into medication management strategies, monitor patient engagement, and provide guidance on their effective use.

Microbiome-based Therapies: The human microbiome plays a crucial role in health and disease. Microbiome-based therapies involve modulating the composition and function of the microbiome to improve patient outcomes. Clinical pharmacists can support microbiome-based therapies by managing medications that interact with the microbiome, monitoring treatment responses, and providing patient education on the role of the microbiome in health and disease.

These emerging therapeutic approaches have the potential to transform healthcare and improve patient outcomes. With their medication expertise, clinical pharmacists can contribute to the safe and effective use of these therapies, provide patient education, monitor treatment responses, and collaborate with healthcare teams to optimize patient care. Staying abreast of these emerging therapeutic approaches will be essential for clinical pharmacists to provide the highest level of patient-centered care in the future.

10. Clinical Pharmacy in Specialized Areas

Dr. Cyril Sajan

10.1 Oncology Pharmacy

Clinical pharmacy plays a vital role in specialized areas such as oncology pharmacy. Oncology pharmacy focuses on the safe and effective use of medications in cancer treatment and care. Here are critical aspects of clinical pharmacy in oncology:

Chemotherapy Management: Clinical pharmacists in oncology collaborate with healthcare teams to ensure appropriate chemotherapy selection, dosing, and administration. They assess patient-specific factors, such as organ function, comorbidities, and drug interactions, to optimize treatment regimens and minimize toxicity.

Adverse Event Management: Oncology pharmacists monitor and manage chemotherapy-related adverse events, such as nausea, vomiting, neutropenia, and mucositis. They provide supportive care recommendations, dose adjustments, and assist in managing side effects to enhance patient comfort and treatment adherence.

Medication Safety: Clinical pharmacists play a critical role in medication safety in oncology. They review chemotherapy orders, ensure accurate preparation, oversee proper handling, and verify appropriate storage and disposal of hazardous medications. They also contribute to the development of standardized protocols and procedures to enhance medication safety in cancer care.

Drug Information and Education: Oncology pharmacists provide drug information and education to healthcare professionals, patients, and their caregivers. They disseminate up-to-date information on chemotherapy agents, potential side effects, drug interactions, and supportive care measures to promote safe and effective medication use.

Clinical Trials: Clinical pharmacists in oncology often participate in clinical trial teams. They help in the development of trial protocols, ensure regulatory compliance, monitor drug-related adverse events, and provide medication management for participants. Their involvement ensures patient safety and adherence to research protocols.

Palliative Care: In collaboration with palliative care teams, clinical pharmacists in oncology play a crucial role in managing pain and other symptoms in patients with advanced or terminal cancer. They optimize pain medication regimens, assist with opioid conversions, and provide recommendations for managing medication-related side effects.

Supportive Care and Survivorship: Oncology pharmacists contribute to supportive care interventions, including the management of treatment-related symptoms, prevention and management of chemotherapy-induced nausea and vomiting, and addressing long-term side effects. They also provide counseling and support for survivors, addressing medication-related concerns and promoting wellness.

Interprofessional Collaboration: Oncology pharmacists collaborate with various healthcare professionals, including oncologists, nurses, social workers, and palliative care teams. They actively participate in interdisciplinary meetings, tumor boards, and patient care conferences, ensuring effective communication and coordination of care.

Oncology pharmacy is a dynamic and rapidly evolving field. Clinical pharmacists specializing in oncology play a vital role in optimizing cancer treatment outcomes, ensuring medication safety, and providing patient-centered care. Their expertise contributes to the multidisciplinary approach in oncology care, addressing the complex medication needs of cancer patients throughout their treatment journey.

10.2 Critical Care Pharmacy

Clinical pharmacy plays a crucial role in critical care settings, where patients require intensive monitoring and specialized medication management. Critical care pharmacy focuses on optimizing medication therapy for critically ill patients in areas such as intensive care units (ICUs) and emergency departments. Here are key aspects of clinical pharmacy in critical care:

Medication Management and Optimization: Clinical pharmacists in critical care collaborate with healthcare teams to assess patients' medication needs and optimize therapy. They ensure appropriate medication selection, dosing, and administration, taking into account factors such as organ function, drug interactions, and pharmacokinetic considerations in critically ill patients.

Pharmacokinetics and Dosing Adjustments: Critical care pharmacists employ pharmacokinetic principles to individualize medication dosing in critically ill patients. They calculate and adjust dosages based on factors like renal and hepatic function, fluid shifts, and altered drug metabolism in the critically ill population.

Sedation and Analgesia Management: Clinical pharmacists are key in managing sedation and analgesia in critically ill patients. They assess pain levels, administer appropriate pain medications, and monitor the effectiveness and side effects of sedatives and analgesics to ensure optimal pain management and patient comfort.

Antimicrobial Stewardship: Critical care pharmacists are actively involved in antimicrobial stewardship programs. They collaborate with infectious disease specialists and other healthcare professionals to optimize antibiotic therapy, prevent the development of antimicrobial resistance, and reduce the incidence of healthcare-associated infections.

Continuous Infusion Medications: Critical care patients often require continuous infusion medications, such as vasoactive agents, sedatives, and antiepileptics. Clinical pharmacists manage these medications, monitor their effects, and make dose adjustments based on patients' hemodynamic stability, sedation levels, and seizure control.

TPN and Parenteral Nutrition: Clinical pharmacists in critical care are responsible for managing total parenteral nutrition (TPN) and other forms of parenteral nutrition. They assess patients' nutritional needs, formulate appropriate TPN regimens, monitor nutritional parameters, and adjust therapy to optimize patients' nutritional status.

Resuscitation and Emergency Medications: Critical care pharmacists are proficient in resuscitation procedures and emergency medication management. They provide immediate access to emergency medications, ensure their appropriate storage and availability, and assist healthcare teams in medication administration during critical situations.

Interprofessional Collaboration: Critical care pharmacists work closely with physicians, nurses, respiratory therapists, and other healthcare professionals in a multidisciplinary team. They actively participate in rounds, contribute to treatment decisions, provide drug information, and assist in optimizing patient care through effective communication and collaboration.

Clinical pharmacy in critical care settings is essential for optimizing medication therapy, ensuring patient safety, and improving outcomes in critically ill patients. Clinical pharmacists' specialized knowledge and expertise in critical care contribute to the comprehensive and coordinated care of critically ill patients, enhancing medication efficacy, minimizing adverse events, and promoting patient recovery.

10.3 Pediatric Pharmacy

Clinical pharmacy in pediatric settings plays a critical role in optimizing medication therapy for children, ensuring safe and effective use of medications. Pediatric pharmacy focuses on the unique medication needs of infants, children, and adolescents. Here are key aspects of clinical pharmacy in pediatric settings:

Pediatric Dosing and Formulations: Clinical pharmacists in pediatric pharmacy calculate and recommend appropriate medication dosages based on the child's weight, age, and developmental stage. They consider factors such as organ maturation, pharmacokinetics, and safety profiles to ensure accurate dosing. Additionally, they collaborate with healthcare teams and compounding pharmacists to prepare specialized formulations suitable for pediatric patients.

Medication Safety and Adverse Event Management: Pediatric pharmacists prioritize medication safety in children. They monitor for adverse drug reactions, drug interactions, and medication errors specific to the pediatric population. They provide guidance on managing medication-related side effects and collaborate with healthcare teams to minimize potential risks.

Neonatal Pharmacy: Clinical pharmacists specializing in neonatal pharmacy provide medication management for critically ill premature infants and newborns. They consider unique challenges such as organ immaturity, variable drug response, and dosing adjustments in this vulnerable population. They work closely with neonatologists and nurses to ensure optimal pharmacotherapy and medication safety.

Pediatric Oncology Pharmacy: Clinical pharmacists in pediatric oncology collaborate with healthcare teams to optimize medication therapy for children with cancer. They assess drug interactions, monitor for chemotherapy-related adverse events, and manage supportive care medications. They also contribute to the management of pain, nausea, and other treatment-related side effects in pediatric oncology patients.

Pediatric Asthma and Allergy Management: Pediatric pharmacists play a role in the management of asthma and allergies in children. They provide education on inhaler techniques, assist in selecting appropriate medications, and monitor treatment responses. They also work with healthcare teams to develop asthma action plans and provide counseling on allergen avoidance and emergency treatment.

Medication Counseling and Education: Pediatric pharmacists provide medication counseling and education to parents and caregivers. They explain medication instructions, dosing schedules, potential side effects, and the importance of medication adherence in a child-friendly and age-appropriate manner. They also address any concerns or questions regarding medications.

Growth and Development Considerations: Clinical pharmacists in pediatric pharmacy consider the impact of medications on a child's growth and development. They monitor growth parameters, evaluate potential effects of long-term medication use, and collaborate with healthcare teams to ensure optimal medication choices that minimize any negative impacts on growth and development.

Interprofessional Collaboration: Pediatric pharmacists work closely with pediatricians, nurses, nutritionists, and other healthcare professionals to provide comprehensive care to children. They actively participate in rounds, contribute to treatment decisions, and provide drug information and expertise to support optimal medication management in pediatric patients.

Clinical pharmacy in pediatric settings requires specialized knowledge, expertise, and a patient-centered approach. Pharmacists play a crucial role in ensuring safe and effective medication therapy for children, collaborating with healthcare teams, and educating patients and caregivers. By providing evidence-based medication management, pediatric pharmacists contribute to improved health outcomes and quality of life for pediatric patients.

10.4 Geriatric Pharmacy

Clinical pharmacy in geriatric settings focuses on optimizing medication therapy for older adults, who often have complex medication regimens and unique healthcare needs. Geriatric pharmacy is crucial in promoting medication safety, reducing adverse drug events, and improving overall health outcomes in older adults. Here are critical aspects of clinical pharmacy in geriatric settings:

Comprehensive Medication Reviews: Geriatric pharmacists conduct comprehensive medication reviews to assess the appropriateness, effectiveness, and safety of medication regimens in older adults. They evaluate potential drug interactions, polypharmacy issues, and medication-related risks, considering age-related physiological changes and comorbidities.

Medication Optimization and Deprescribing: Clinical pharmacists collaborate with healthcare teams to optimize medication therapy in older adults. They identify opportunities for deprescribing and minimizing unnecessary or inappropriate medications, considering factors such as the potential for adverse effects, limited life expectancy, and patient goals of care. They work closely with healthcare providers to adjust dosages, simplify regimens, and promote medication adherence.

Geriatric-Specific Conditions: Geriatric pharmacists specialize in managing medications for age-related conditions prevalent in older adults, such as cognitive decline, osteoporosis, urinary incontinence, and chronic pain. They provide recommendations on appropriate medications, dosing adjustments, and monitoring strategies for optimal management of these conditions.

Fall Prevention and Medication Safety: Geriatric pharmacists play a vital role in fall prevention and medication safety in older adults. They identify medications that may increase the risk of falls and collaborate with healthcare teams to minimize fall hazards. They also provide education on medication-related fall prevention strategies and assist in managing medication-related side effects that may impact mobility and balance.

Polypharmacy Management: Clinical pharmacists in geriatric settings address the challenges of polypharmacy, where older adults are taking multiple medications. They evaluate medication appropriateness, optimize regimens to minimize drug interactions and adverse effects, and provide patient education on medication schedules and potential side effects.

Age-Related Pharmacokinetics and Pharmacodynamics: Geriatric pharmacists consider age-related changes in pharmacokinetics and pharmacodynamics when managing medications for older adults. They account for altered drug absorption, distribution, metabolism, and elimination in this population. By considering individualized medication regimens, they optimize treatment outcomes while minimizing the risk of adverse effects.

Interprofessional Collaboration: Geriatric pharmacists collaborate with a multidisciplinary team, including geriatricians, primary care physicians, nurses, and social workers, to provide comprehensive care to older adults. They actively participate in interprofessional meetings, medication reconciliation processes, and care conferences to ensure coordinated and patient-centered care.

Medication Adherence Support: Geriatric pharmacists assist older adults in adhering to their medication regimens. They provide counseling on medication use, address barriers to adherence (e.g., cognitive impairment, physical limitations), and recommend strategies to enhance medication adherence, such as pill organizers or reminder systems.

Clinical pharmacy in geriatric settings requires specialized knowledge in geriatric pharmacotherapy, age-related considerations, and medication management for older adults. Pharmacists play a vital role in promoting medication safety, optimizing therapy, and improving the quality of life for older adults by addressing their unique medication-related needs.

10.5 Ambulatory Care Pharmacy

Clinical pharmacy in ambulatory care settings focuses on providing patient-centered care in outpatient settings, such as clinics, community pharmacies, and primary care practices. Ambulatory care pharmacists work collaboratively with healthcare teams to optimize medication therapy and improve patient outcomes. Here are key aspects of clinical pharmacy in ambulatory care:

Medication Therapy Management: Ambulatory care pharmacists perform comprehensive medication reviews and assessments to optimize medication therapy. They work with patients to identify medication-related issues, ensure appropriate medication selection, dosing, and adherence, and monitor treatment responses.

Chronic Disease Management: Ambulatory care pharmacists play a crucial role in managing chronic diseases, such as diabetes, hypertension, asthma, and cardiovascular conditions. They educate patients, develop individualized care plans, monitor medication effectiveness and side effects, and help patients achieve treatment goals.

Medication Adherence Support: Ambulatory care pharmacists assist patients in adhering to their medication regimens. They provide counseling on medication use, address barriers to adherence, offer adherence aids (e.g., pill organizers, reminder systems), and collaborate with patients to develop strategies for successful medication adherence.

Preventive Care and Health Promotion: Ambulatory care pharmacists contribute to preventive care and health promotion initiatives. They provide immunizations, conduct screenings (e.g., blood pressure, cholesterol), and offer counseling on lifestyle modifications (e.g., smoking cessation, weight management) to promote overall health and disease prevention.

Transitions of Care: Ambulatory care pharmacists facilitate smooth care transitions between different healthcare settings. They ensure the continuity of medication therapy, reconcile medication lists, and educate patients on medication changes when transitioning from hospital to home or between healthcare providers.

Collaborative Practice and Interprofessional Care: Ambulatory care pharmacists actively collaborate with healthcare teams, including physicians, nurses, and other healthcare professionals. They participate in interprofessional meetings, contribute to care planning, provide drug information and expertise, and ensure coordinated and comprehensive patient care.

Medication Cost Management: Ambulatory care pharmacists help patients navigate medication costs and access affordable treatment options. They provide information on drug pricing, assistance programs, and therapeutic alternatives to improve medication affordability and reduce financial barriers to adherence.

Specialty Medication Management: Ambulatory care pharmacists may specialize in managing complex medications, such as biologics, specialty drugs, and high-cost therapies. They provide counseling on medication administration, monitor treatment response, assess for side effects, and ensure appropriate medication access and adherence.

Ambulatory care pharmacists are positioned to provide accessible, patient-centered care in outpatient settings. Their expertise in medication therapy management, chronic disease management, and preventive care contributes to improved patient outcomes and enhanced medication safety in ambulatory care settings. Ambulatory care pharmacists work collaboratively with healthcare teams to optimize medication therapy and promote overall health and well-being.

11. Challenges and Opportunities for Clinical Pharmacists

Dr. Cyril Sajan

11.1 Regulatory and Legal Considerations

Clinical pharmacists face several challenges and opportunities related to regulatory and legal considerations. These considerations impact their ability to provide optimal patient care and contribute to the evolving healthcare landscape. Here are key challenges and opportunities in regulatory and legal aspects for clinical pharmacists:

Challenges:

Scope of Practice Restrictions: Clinical pharmacists may face scope of practice restrictions imposed by regulatory bodies or state laws. These restrictions can limit their ability to utilize their expertise and contribute to patient care fully.

Licensure and Credentialing: Clinical pharmacists may encounter challenges related to licensure and credentialing. Obtaining and maintaining appropriate licensure and credentials, including board certifications, can be time-consuming and involve complex processes.

Collaborative Practice Agreements: Some states require clinical pharmacists to establish collective practice agreements with physicians or other healthcare providers. Developing and maintaining these agreements can present administrative burdens and vary across practice settings and jurisdictions.

Reimbursement and Payment Models: Clinical pharmacists may face challenges securing appropriate reimbursement for their services. The lack of standardized reimbursement mechanisms and limited recognition of clinical pharmacy services can hinder their ability to provide comprehensive patient care.

Formulary Restrictions and Access to Medications: Clinical pharmacists may face formulary restrictions imposed by insurance providers, which can impact patient access to certain medications. Working within formulary constraints requires proactive communication with healthcare teams to identify alternatives and advocate for patient needs.

Opportunities:

Expansion of Clinical Pharmacy Services: There is an increasing recognition of clinical pharmacists' value to the healthcare team. Opportunities exist to expand clinical pharmacy services and integrate pharmacists into new practice settings, such as primary care clinics, specialty clinics, and outpatient care centers.

Collaborative Practice and Team-Based Care: The shift towards collaborative practice models and team-based care presents opportunities for clinical pharmacists to work closely with other healthcare professionals. Collaborative practice allows for improved patient outcomes, better utilization of pharmacist expertise, and enhanced interprofessional collaboration.

Advancement of Provider Status: Clinical pharmacists have been advocating for recognition as healthcare providers at the federal and state levels. Provider status would grant them greater autonomy, expanded scope of practice, and improved service reimbursement.

Implementation of Practice Guidelines and Protocols: Developing and implementing practice guidelines and protocols specific to clinical pharmacy can enhance the standardization of care and ensure consistent delivery of evidence-based practice across different healthcare settings.

Integration of Technology: Technological advancements, such as electronic health records, telehealth platforms, and digital health applications, offer opportunities for clinical pharmacists to streamline their workflows, enhance communication, and provide remote patient care services.

Advocacy and Professional Organizations: Clinical pharmacists can leverage professional organizations and advocacy efforts to influence regulatory and legal considerations. Active involvement in these organizations can help shape policies, regulations, and legislation that impact clinical pharmacy practice.

Navigating the regulatory and legal landscape is crucial for clinical pharmacists to provide high-quality patient care and maximize their impact within the healthcare system. By seizing opportunities and addressing challenges, clinical pharmacists can continue to evolve their practice and contribute to improving patient outcomes.

11.2 Education and Training

Clinical pharmacists face various challenges and opportunities related to education and training. These factors significantly impact their ability to provide quality patient care and adapt to the evolving healthcare landscape. Here are key challenges and opportunities in education and training for clinical pharmacists:

Challenges:

Evolving Knowledge and Skills: The pharmacy field is continuously changing with new medications, treatment guidelines, and technological advancements. Clinical pharmacists must stay updated with the latest evidence-based practices, drug information, and therapeutic procedures to provide optimal patient care.

Continuing Education Requirements: Clinical pharmacists must meet continuing education requirements to maintain their licensure and board certifications. These requirements ensure ongoing professional development but can be time-consuming and challenging to fulfill while balancing work responsibilities.

Training Opportunities: Clinical pharmacists may face challenges accessing diverse training opportunities to enhance their skills and expand their knowledge base. Availability and access to specialized training programs, preceptorships, and fellowships can vary based on geographic location and practice settings.

Interprofessional Education: Collaborative practice and interprofessional care are essential in modern healthcare. Clinical pharmacists need opportunities for interprofessional education and training to develop effective communication, teamwork, and collaboration skills.

Limited Residency Positions: Securing a residency position is highly competitive, and the number of available positions may not meet the demand. The limited availability of residency training can make it challenging for clinical pharmacists to gain specialized clinical experience and enhance their clinical skills.

Opportunities:

Advanced Training and Specialization: Clinical pharmacists can pursue advanced training and specialization through postgraduate residency programs, fellowships, and specialized certifications. These opportunities allow pharmacists to gain in-depth knowledge and expertise in specific areas, such as critical care, oncology, or ambulatory care.

PharmD Curriculum Enhancement: Pharmacy schools have the opportunity to enhance the Doctor of Pharmacy (PharmD) curriculum to incorporate more clinical and patient-centered education. This includes integrating interprofessional education, pharmacogenomics, evidence-based medicine, and clinical decision-making skills.

Collaboration with Academic Institutions: Clinical pharmacists can collaborate with academic institutions as preceptors and adjunct faculty members. Involvement in academia allows pharmacists to contribute to the education and training of future pharmacists, engage in research, and stay connected to the latest advancements in the field.

Continuing Professional Development: Clinical pharmacists can take advantage of various continuing professional development opportunities, such as conferences, workshops, webinars, and online courses. These resources enable pharmacists to stay updated with the latest research, guidelines, and clinical practices.

Leadership and Mentorship Roles: Clinical pharmacists have opportunities to take on leadership and mentorship roles within their organizations or professional associations. By serving as mentors, preceptors, or leaders, pharmacists can contribute to the development and growth of future pharmacists and promote the advancement of the profession.

Integration of Technology in Education: The integration of technology, such as online learning platforms, simulation tools, and virtual patient encounters, offers innovative ways to enhance education and training for clinical pharmacists. These technologies facilitate interactive learning, case-based scenarios, and self-assessment, allowing pharmacists to develop and refine their clinical skills.

Lifelong Learning: Lifelong learning is a fundamental aspect of the pharmacy profession. Clinical pharmacists have the opportunity to embrace lifelong learning by actively seeking new knowledge, engaging in self-directed learning, and staying curious and open to new experiences.

Continual education and training are essential for clinical pharmacists to maintain competence, expand their skills, and adapt to the changing healthcare landscape. By embracing opportunities for advanced training, engaging in interprofessional education, and actively pursuing continuing education, clinical pharmacists can provide high-quality patient care and drive advancements in the field.

11.3 Advancement and Recognition

Clinical pharmacists face various challenges and opportunities related to education and training. These factors significantly impact their ability to provide quality patient care and adapt to the evolving healthcare landscape. Here are key challenges and opportunities in education and training for clinical pharmacists:

Challenges:

Evolving Knowledge and Skills: The pharmacy field is continuously changing with new medications, treatment guidelines, and technological advancements. Clinical pharmacists must stay updated with the latest evidence-based practices, drug information, and therapeutic procedures to provide optimal patient care.

Continuing Education Requirements: Clinical pharmacists must meet continuing education requirements to maintain their licensure and board certifications. These requirements ensure ongoing professional development but can be time-consuming and challenging to fulfill while balancing work responsibilities.

Training Opportunities: Clinical pharmacists may face challenges accessing diverse training opportunities to enhance their skills and expand their knowledge base. Availability and access to specialized training programs, preceptorships, and fellowships can vary based on geographic location and practice settings.

Interprofessional Education: Collaborative practice and interprofessional care are essential in modern healthcare. Clinical pharmacists need opportunities for interprofessional education and training to develop effective communication, teamwork, and collaboration skills.

Limited Residency Positions: Securing a residency position is highly competitive, and the number of available positions may need to meet the demand. The limited availability of residency training can make it challenging for clinical pharmacists to gain specialized clinical experience and enhance their clinical skills.

Opportunities:

Advanced Training and Specialization: Clinical pharmacists can pursue advanced training and specialization through postgraduate residency programs, fellowships, and specialized certifications. These opportunities allow pharmacists to gain in-depth knowledge and expertise in specific areas, such as critical care, oncology, or ambulatory care.

PharmD Curriculum Enhancement: Pharmacy schools have the opportunity to enhance the Doctor of Pharmacy (PharmD) curriculum to incorporate more clinical and patient-centered education. This includes integrating interprofessional education, pharmacogenomics, evidence-based medicine, and clinical decision-making skills.

Collaboration with Academic Institutions: Clinical pharmacists can collaborate with academic institutions as preceptors and adjunct faculty members. Involvement in academia allows pharmacists to contribute to the education and training of future pharmacists, engage in research, and stay connected to the latest advancements in the field.

Continuing Professional Development: Clinical pharmacists can use various continuing professional development opportunities, such as conferences, workshops, webinars, and online courses. These resources enable pharmacists to stay updated with the latest research, guidelines, and clinical practices.

Leadership and Mentorship Roles: Clinical pharmacists have opportunities to take on leadership and mentorship roles within their organizations or professional associations. By serving as mentors, preceptors, or leaders, pharmacists can contribute to the development and growth of future pharmacists and promote the profession's advancement.

Integration of Technology in Education: Integrating technology, such as online learning platforms, simulation tools, and virtual patient encounters, offers innovative ways to enhance education and training for clinical pharmacists. These technologies facilitate interactive learning, case-based scenarios, and self-assessment, allowing pharmacists to develop and refine their clinical skills.

Lifelong Learning: Lifelong learning is a fundamental aspect of the pharmacy profession. Clinical pharmacists can embrace lifelong learning by actively seeking new knowledge, engaging in self-directed learning, and staying curious and open to new experiences.

Continual education and training are essential for clinical pharmacists to maintain competence, expand their skills, and adapt to the changing healthcare landscape. By embracing opportunities for advanced training, engaging in interprofessional education, and actively pursuing continuing education, clinical pharmacists can provide high-quality patient care and drive advancements in the field.

11.4 Collaboration and Communication

Clinical pharmacists face various challenges and opportunities in collaboration and communication within interprofessional healthcare teams. Effective collaboration and communication are essential for providing comprehensive patient care and optimizing medication therapy outcomes. Here are key challenges and opportunities in collaboration and communication for clinical pharmacists:

Challenges:

Lack of Understanding of Clinical Pharmacist Role: Some healthcare professionals may need more knowledge and understanding of the clinical pharmacist's scope of practice and the value they bring to the healthcare team. This can create barriers to effective collaboration and limit opportunities for clinical pharmacists to contribute fully to patient care.

Hierarchical Structures and Communication Barriers: Hierarchical structures within healthcare settings can create communication barriers, making it challenging for clinical pharmacists to communicate their recommendations and concerns to other healthcare professionals effectively. Overcoming these barriers requires fostering a culture of open communication and mutual respect.

Limited Interprofessional Education: Interprofessional education opportunities during training programs may be limited, leading to inadequate preparation for collaborative practice. With a solid foundation in interprofessional collaboration, clinical pharmacists may be able to effectively communicate and collaborate with other healthcare professionals.

Time Constraints: Healthcare professionals, including clinical pharmacists, often face time constraints in their practice settings. Limited face-to-face communication and collaboration time can hinder effective information exchange, care coordination, and decision-making.

Opportunities:

Interprofessional Collaboration Models: Embracing interprofessional collaboration models, such as collaborative drug therapy management and team-based care, creates opportunities for clinical pharmacists to work alongside other healthcare professionals in a coordinated and cooperative manner. These models enhance communication and allow for the sharing of expertise and responsibilities.

Communication Skills Training: Clinical pharmacists can enhance communication skills through training programs and workshops. Practical communication skills, such as active listening, clear and concise messaging, and conflict resolution, enable pharmacists to effectively convey their recommendations, address concerns, and build strong relationships with other healthcare professionals.

Interprofessional Education and Training: Incorporating interprofessional education and training into pharmacy curricula and continuing education programs helps prepare clinical pharmacists for effective collaboration. Experiential learning opportunities, case-based discussions, and interprofessional simulation exercises foster teamwork and communication skills among healthcare professionals.

Participation in Interdisciplinary Rounds and Meetings: Participating in interdisciplinary rounds, team meetings, and care conferences provides clinical pharmacists with opportunities to share their expertise, contribute to treatment decisions, and engage in collaborative problem-solving. Regular participation enhances their visibility and strengthens relationships with other healthcare professionals.

Electronic Health Records and Communication Platforms: Utilizing electronic health records (EHRs) and communication platforms, such as secure messaging systems, facilitates timely and efficient communication between clinical pharmacists and other healthcare team members. Access to shared patient information improves coordination and promotes collaborative decision-making.

Shared Decision-Making: Shared decision-making with patients and healthcare professionals fosters collaboration and strengthens relationships. Clinical pharmacists can actively involve patients in medication-related decisions and collaborate with other healthcare professionals to ensure patient-centered care.

Professional Networking: Networking with other healthcare professionals through professional organizations, conferences, and local events creates collaboration and relationship building opportunities. Building a solid professional network enables clinical pharmacists to engage in interdisciplinary collaborations and stay connected with the broader healthcare community.

Efficient collaboration and effective communication are crucial for clinical pharmacists to contribute fully to interprofessional healthcare teams. By embracing collaborative models, enhancing communication skills, participating in interdisciplinary activities, and leveraging technology, clinical pharmacists can overcome challenges and seize opportunities to provide optimal patient care and improve medication therapy outcomes.

11.5 Advocacy and Leadership

Clinical pharmacists face various challenges and opportunities related to advocacy and leadership within the healthcare system. Advocacy and leadership are crucial for advancing the profession, influencing policy changes, and promoting optimal patient care. Here are key challenges and opportunities in advocacy and leadership for clinical pharmacists:

Challenges:

Limited Awareness of Clinical Pharmacy: One of the challenges is the need for more awareness among healthcare professionals, policymakers, and the general public regarding the role and value of clinical pharmacists in patient care. This lack of understanding can hinder the recognition and integration of clinical pharmacists into healthcare teams.

Fragmented Advocacy Efforts: Advocacy efforts within the pharmacy profession may need to be more cohesive, with individual practitioners and professional organizations advocating independently. This fragmentation can reduce the collective impact and effectiveness of advocacy initiatives.

Influence of External Stakeholders: Clinical pharmacists face challenges in navigating the result of external stakeholders, such as insurance providers, regulatory bodies, and pharmaceutical companies, on policy decisions and healthcare practices. Aligning these external stakeholders' interests with the goals of clinical pharmacy practice can be challenging.

Limited Leadership Opportunities: Clinical pharmacists may need more opportunities for leadership roles within their organizations or professional associations. This limitation can hinder their ability to drive change, shape policies, and advocate for the profession's advancement.

Opportunities:

Professional Organizations and Associations: Clinical pharmacists can actively engage with organizations and associations dedicated to advancing the profession. Joining and participating in these groups provide opportunities to contribute to advocacy efforts, shape policy decisions, and collaborate with like-minded professionals.

Legislative and Policy Advocacy: Clinical pharmacists can engage in legislative advocacy by participating in grassroots campaigns, contacting elected officials, and educating policymakers about the value of clinical pharmacy services. They can also collaborate with professional organizations to influence policy changes that positively impact patient care and the profession.

Patient Advocacy: Advocating for patient-centered care is a powerful way for clinical pharmacists to promote the profession. By actively engaging with patients, educating them about their medications, and advocating for their needs, clinical pharmacists can demonstrate their value in improving patient outcomes.

Leadership Development Programs: Clinical pharmacists can use leadership development programs and workshops to enhance their leadership skills. These programs provide the knowledge and skills necessary for clinical pharmacists to effectively lead teams, drive change, and influence healthcare practices.

Research and Publication: Clinical pharmacists can contribute to the profession's advancement by conducting research, publishing findings in reputable journals, and presenting at conferences. Evidence-based research strengthens the credibility of clinical pharmacists and provides a platform for advocacy and leadership in the field.

Collaborative Partnerships: Building collaborative partnerships with other healthcare professionals, patient advocacy groups, and industry stakeholders can amplify the voice and influence of clinical pharmacists. Collaborative efforts allow for shared advocacy goals and a more substantial collective impact on advancing patient care and the profession.

Public Awareness Campaigns: Clinical pharmacists can engage in public awareness campaigns to educate the public about the role and impact of clinical pharmacy. By raising awareness of their contributions to patient care and medication safety, clinical pharmacists can garner support and recognition from the public and policymakers.

Advocacy and leadership are essential for clinical pharmacists to shape the profession's future and contribute to optimal patient care. By actively engaging in advocacy initiatives, developing leadership skills, and collaborating with others, clinical pharmacists can overcome challenges and seize opportunities to advocate for their profession, influence policy decisions, and drive positive change in the healthcare system.

12. Conclusion

Dr. Hemraj Singh Rajput, Dr. Rajesh Hadia, Dr. Varun Singh Saggu, Dr. Cyril Sajan

12.1 Summary of Key Findings

In conclusion, this exploration of the evolving landscape of clinical pharmacy has highlighted several key findings:

- ✓ Clinical pharmacy has evolved from focusing on dispensing medications to a patient-centered approach that emphasizes optimizing medication therapy and improving patient outcomes.
- ✓ The role of clinical pharmacists has expanded to include medication therapy management, pharmaceutical care, drug information services, clinical decision support systems, and medication reconciliation.
- ✓ Technological advances, such as electronic health records, telepharmacy, clinical pharmacy software, and pharmacy automation systems, have revolutionized clinical pharmacy practice, enhancing efficiency and patient care.
- ✓ Precision medicine and personalized pharmacotherapy, driven by genomics, pharmacogenomics, and biomarkers, are transforming how medications are prescribed and individualized treatment approaches are developed.
- ✓ Integration of pharmacists in interprofessional healthcare teams has become increasingly important, contributing to improved patient outcomes through collaborative practice models, team-based care, and effective communication.
- ✓ Emerging roles for clinical pharmacists, including pharmacogeneticists, pharmacovigilance specialists, clinical pharmacy consultants, transitions of care pharmacists, and clinical research pharmacists, offer new opportunities for specialization and enhanced patient care.

- ✓ Contemporary issues in clinical pharmacy, such as medication safety and quality assurance, drug pricing and affordability, pharmaceutical industry influence, medication adherence challenges, and global health and access to medicines, present ongoing challenges and areas for improvement.
- ✓ Future perspectives in clinical pharmacy, including artificial intelligence and machine learning, virtual and augmented reality, nanotechnology in drug delivery, blockchain technology, and emerging therapeutic approaches, are promising for advancing patient care and medication management.
- ✓ Clinical pharmacy in specialized areas, such as oncology pharmacy, critical care pharmacy, pediatric pharmacy, geriatric pharmacy, and ambulatory care pharmacy, requires specialized knowledge and skills to address the unique needs of patients in these settings.
- ✓ Challenges and opportunities for clinical pharmacists in areas such as regulatory and legal considerations, education and training, advancement and recognition, collaboration and communication, and advocacy and leadership shape the profession's future.

Overall, clinical pharmacy continues to evolve, embracing technological advancements, personalized medicine, interdisciplinary collaboration, and patient-centered care. Clinical pharmacists are vital in optimizing medication therapy, ensuring patient safety, and improving healthcare outcomes. As the healthcare landscape continues to change, clinical pharmacists will remain at the forefront of providing evidence-based, personalized care to patients, contributing to the overall quality and effectiveness of healthcare delivery.

12.2 Implications for Clinical Pharmacy Practice

The exploration of the evolving landscape of clinical pharmacy has significant implications for the practice of clinical pharmacists. The key findings shed light on the changing role of clinical pharmacists, technological advancements, personalized pharmacotherapy, interprofessional collaboration, emerging roles, contemporary issues, future perspectives, and specialized areas of practice. These implications shape how clinical pharmacists provide patient care and contribute to the healthcare system.

Firstly, clinical pharmacists must embrace their expanded role as medication therapy experts and patient advocates. They should actively engage in medication therapy management, pharmaceutical care, drug information services, clinical decision support systems, and medication reconciliation to ensure safe and effective medication use.

Secondly, clinical pharmacists must keep up with technological advances in electronic health records, telepharmacy, clinical pharmacy software, and pharmacy automation systems. Integrating these technologies into their practice can enhance efficiency, accuracy, and patient care delivery.

Thirdly, clinical pharmacists should embrace the principles of precision medicine and personalized pharmacotherapy, utilizing genomics, pharmacogenomics, and biomarkers to individualize treatment approaches and optimize medication regimens.

Fourthly, interprofessional collaboration is essential for clinical pharmacists. They should actively participate in healthcare teams, contribute to collaborative practice models, and enhance communication skills to communicate and collaborate with other healthcare professionals effectively.

Fifthly, clinical pharmacists should explore emerging roles such as pharmacogeneticists, pharmacovigilance specialists, clinical pharmacy consultants, transitions of care pharmacists, and clinical research pharmacists. These roles offer opportunities for specialization, advanced practice, and contributing to innovative healthcare initiatives.

Sixthly, clinical pharmacists must address contemporary issues in medication safety and quality assurance, drug pricing and affordability, pharmaceutical industry influence, medication adherence challenges, and global health and access to medicines. They should advocate for patient-centered solutions, contribute to policy changes, and work towards improving healthcare access and affordability.

Seventhly, clinical pharmacists should stay informed about future perspectives in clinical pharmacy, including artificial intelligence and machine learning, virtual reality and augmented reality, nanotechnology in drug delivery, blockchain technology, and emerging therapeutic approaches. Embracing these advancements can enhance their practice and improve patient care outcomes.

Finally, clinical pharmacists in specialized areas such as oncology pharmacy, critical care pharmacy, pediatric pharmacy, geriatric pharmacy, and ambulatory care pharmacy should continuously enhance their knowledge and skills to provide specialized care to patients in these settings.

Overall, the implications for clinical pharmacy practice are diverse and evolving. Clinical pharmacists must adapt to these changes, continuously learn, advocate for their profession, and collaborate with other healthcare professionals to provide patient-centered, evidence-based care. By embracing these implications, clinical pharmacists can positively impact patient outcomes, advance the pharmacy field, and contribute to the overall improvement of the healthcare system.

12.3 Recommendations for Future Research

While exploring the evolving landscape of clinical pharmacy, several areas for future research have emerged. These research recommendations can further enhance the understanding and practice of clinical pharmacy. Here are some key recommendations:

Evaluation of the Impact of Technological Advances: Research to assess the impact of electronic health records, telepharmacy, clinical pharmacy software, pharmacy automation systems, and mobile applications on patient outcomes, medication safety, and pharmacist workflow. Investigate the benefits and challenges associated with implementing these technologies in different healthcare settings.

Assessment of Personalized Pharmacotherapy Approaches: Investigate the effectiveness and cost-effectiveness of personalized pharmacotherapy approaches, such as genomics and pharmacogenomics, in improving medication selection, dosage optimization, and patient outcomes. Explore the barriers and facilitators to implementing personalized pharmacotherapy in clinical practice.

Study the Role of Clinical Pharmacists in Specialized Areas: Research to evaluate the impact of clinical pharmacists in specialized areas, such as oncology pharmacies, critical care pharmacy, pediatric pharmacy, geriatric pharmacy, and ambulatory care pharmacy. Assess their roles, contributions, and outcomes in these settings, and identify best practices for optimizing patient care.

Evaluation of Collaborative Practice Models: Investigate the effectiveness and impact of collaborative practice models involving clinical pharmacists and other healthcare professionals. Assess the outcomes of interprofessional collaboration, communication, and care coordination on patient outcomes, healthcare utilization, and medication-related problems.

Examination of Barriers and Facilitators in Clinical Pharmacy Practice: Identify and explore the barriers and facilitators that clinical pharmacists encounter in their practice, including regulatory and legal considerations, education and training, advancement and recognition, collaboration and communication, and advocacy and leadership. Understand these factors to inform strategies for overcoming challenges and maximizing opportunities for clinical pharmacists.

Assessment of Medication Safety and Quality Assurance: Conduct research to assess the effectiveness of medication safety initiatives and quality assurance programs in clinical pharmacy practice. Investigate the impact of these interventions on medication errors, adverse drug events, and patient outcomes. Explore innovative approaches for improving medication safety and quality assurance in diverse healthcare settings.

Study the Impact of Clinical Pharmacy Interventions on Health Economics: Evaluate the economic impact of clinical pharmacy interventions, such as medication therapy management, on healthcare costs, resource utilization, and patient outcomes. Investigate the cost-effectiveness of clinical pharmacy services and their potential for reducing overall healthcare expenditures.

Examination of Patient Perspectives and Satisfaction: Explore patient perspectives and satisfaction regarding the role of clinical pharmacists in their healthcare. Assess patient experiences, perceptions of medication-related care, and the impact of clinical pharmacy services on their medication adherence, quality of life, and overall satisfaction with healthcare.

Investigation of Emerging Technologies and Therapeutic Approaches: Research the applications and implications of emerging technologies, such as artificial intelligence, virtual reality, augmented reality, nanotechnology, and blockchain, in clinical pharmacy practice. Evaluate their potential to enhance medication therapy management, patient engagement, and healthcare outcomes.

Longitudinal Studies on the Career Trajectories of Clinical Pharmacists: Conduct longitudinal studies to understand clinical pharmacists' career trajectories, professional development, and job satisfaction. Investigate the factors influencing career advancement, leadership opportunities, and the impact of expanded roles on professional growth and job satisfaction.

By conducting research in these areas, the field of clinical pharmacy can continue to evolve, inform evidence-based practice, and contribute to improving patient care. These research recommendations can advance the understanding of clinical pharmacy practice, guide policy decisions, and inform educational initiatives to enhance the role of clinical pharmacists in the healthcare system.

References

- American College of Clinical Pharmacy (ACCP): www.accp.com
- American Society of Health-System Pharmacists (ASHP): www.ashp.org
- International Pharmaceutical Federation (FIP): www.fip.org
- The Journal of Clinical Pharmacy and Therapeutics
- Pharmacotherapy: The Journal of Human Pharmacology and Drug Therapy
- Clinical Pharmacology & Therapeutics
- Journal of the American Pharmacists Association
- World Health Organization (WHO) Medication Safety Program: www.who.int/medicines/areas/quality_safety/safety_efficacy/emp_mes/en/
- Institute for Safe Medication Practices (ISMP): www.ismp.org
- American Society of Clinical Oncology (ASCO): www.asco.org
- Society of Critical Care Medicine (SCCM): www.sccm.org
- American Academy of Pediatrics (AAP): www.aap.org
- American Geriatrics Society (AGS): www.americangeriatrics.org
- American Pharmacists Association (APhA): www.pharmacist.com
- Accreditation Council for Pharmacy Education (ACPE): www.acpe-accredit.org

Appendix

Dr. Hemraj Singh Rajput, Dr. Rajesh Hadia, Dr. Varun Singh Saggu, Dr. Cyril Sajan

Appendix A: Glossary of Terms

1. Clinical Pharmacy: A discipline of pharmacy that focuses on the rational use of medications, optimizing medication therapy outcomes, and improving patient care.

2. Medication Therapy Management (MTM): A comprehensive approach to patient care that involves optimizing medication use, ensuring medication safety, and improving medication-related outcomes through medication review, patient education, and collaborative decision-making.

3. Pharmaceutical Care: A patient-centered practice that involves medication therapy management, pharmaceutical consultation, and medication counseling to ensure safe and effective medication use.

4. Drug Information Services: Services provided by clinical pharmacists to gather, evaluate, and disseminate drug-related information to healthcare professionals, patients, and other stakeholders.

5. Clinical Decision Support Systems: Computer-based systems provide healthcare professionals with evidence-based recommendations, alerts, and information to support clinical decision-making and improve patient care.

6. Medication Reconciliation: Creating a complete and accurate list of a patient's medications and comparing it with the medication orders to identify discrepancies, ensure appropriate medication use, and prevent medication errors.

7. Electronic Health Records (EHRs): Digital records that contain comprehensive and up-to-date information about a patient's health, including medical history, diagnoses, medications, lab results, and treatment plans.

8. Telepharmacy: Providing pharmaceutical care and medication-related services through telecommunications technology, enabling remote access to pharmacists and medication expertise.

9. Clinical Pharmacy Software: Software applications designed to support clinical pharmacy practice, including medication management, drug interaction checking, clinical documentation, and data analysis.

10. Pharmacy Automation Systems: Automated systems used in pharmacies to streamline medication dispensing, inventory management, prescription filling, and medication packaging, enhancing accuracy and efficiency.

11. Genomics: The study of an individual's complete set of DNA, including the genes and their functions, and how they influence health and disease.

12. Pharmacogenomics: The study of how an individual's genetic makeup influences their medication response, including drug metabolism, efficacy, and adverse reactions.

13. Biomarkers: Measurable characteristics or indicators that can be used to assess normal biological processes, disease states, or responses to therapy. In clinical decision-making, biomarkers can help guide treatment choices and monitor treatment effectiveness.

14. Interprofessional Healthcare Teams: Collaborative teams that include healthcare professionals from different disciplines working together to provide comprehensive and coordinated patient care.

15. Precision Medicine: An approach to healthcare that considers individual variability in genes, environment, and lifestyle to tailor medical treatments to specific patients or patient subgroups.

16. Personalized Pharmacotherapy: Individualized treatment approaches that consider a patient's unique characteristics, including their genetic makeup, biomarker status, and clinical presentation, to optimize medication selection, dosage, and treatment outcomes.

17. Blockchain Technology: A decentralized, secure, and transparent digital ledger that records and verifies transactions, providing a safe and tamper-proof platform for managing pharmaceutical supply chains, tracking medication authenticity, and improving medication safety.

18. Artificial Intelligence (AI) and Machine Learning: Technologies that enable computer systems to perform tasks that typically require human intelligence, such as data analysis, pattern recognition, and decision-making, to support clinical decision support systems and enhance medication management.

19. Virtual Reality (VR) and Augmented Reality (AR): Technologies that create immersive and interactive virtual environments (VR) or overlay digital information on the real world (AR), with potential applications in healthcare education, training, and patient engagement.

20. Nanotechnology in Drug Delivery: The application of nanoscale materials and techniques to design and deliver medications, enabling targeted drug delivery, improved drug efficacy, and reduced side effects.

21. Clinical Research Pharmacists: Pharmacists who specialize in conducting and overseeing clinical research studies, including clinical trials, to evaluate medication safety, efficacy, and effectiveness.

22. Medication Safety: The prevention of medication errors, adverse drug events, and patient harm resulting from medication use.

23. Drug Pricing and Affordability: Concerns related to the cost of medications and access to affordable medicines, including the impact on patient's ability to obtain needed treatments and healthcare systems' ability to provide sustainable and equitable care.

24. Pharmaceutical Industry Influence: The influence of pharmaceutical companies on healthcare practices, drug development, marketing, and prescribing patterns, and the potential impact on patient care, medication access, and healthcare costs.

25. Medication Adherence: The extent to which patients take their medications as prescribed, including factors influencing adherence, interventions to improve compliance, and the impact on treatment outcomes.

26. Global Health and Access to Medicines: Concerns related to equitable access to essential medications and healthcare services worldwide, including challenges in low-income countries, medication shortages, and disparities in healthcare access and affordability.

27. Regulatory and Legal Considerations: The laws, regulations, and guidelines that govern the practice of clinical pharmacy, including licensure requirements, scope of course, and pharmacist prescribing authority.

28. Education and Training: The educational requirements, curricula, and training programs that prepare pharmacists for clinical pharmacy practice, including continuing education and advanced training opportunities.

29. Advocacy and Leadership: Activities aimed at promoting the role and value of clinical pharmacists, influencing policy decisions, and driving positive changes in healthcare systems, as well as the

development of leadership skills to lead and advance the profession effectively.

Appendix B: Examples of Clinical Pharmacy Practice Models

- ➢ Collaborative Drug Therapy Management (CDTM) Model: In this model, clinical pharmacists work collaboratively with other healthcare providers, such as physicians or nurse practitioners, to manage and adjust patient medication therapy. Clinical pharmacists have the authority to initiate, modify, or discontinue medications under agreed-upon protocols and collaborative agreements.
- ➢ Ambulatory Care Model: Clinical pharmacists provide direct patient care in outpatient settings, such as clinics or primary care practices. They perform medication therapy management, conduct comprehensive medication reviews, provide patient education, monitor treatment outcomes, and collaborate with other healthcare professionals to optimize medication therapy.
- ➢ Transitions of Care Model: Clinical pharmacists play a vital role in ensuring safe and effective transitions of care for patients moving between different healthcare settings, such as hospitals, nursing homes, and home care. They reconcile medication lists, identify and resolve discrepancies, provide medication counseling, and collaborate with healthcare teams to prevent medication-related problems during transitions.
- ➢ Clinical Pharmacy Consultation Model: Clinical pharmacists provide specialized medication expertise and consultation services to healthcare teams. They review medication orders, make recommendations for appropriate therapy, provide drug information, and assist in medication management decisions. This model is often used in hospitals and specialized healthcare settings.

- Telepharmacy Model: In this model, clinical pharmacists provide remote pharmaceutical care services through telecommunication technology. They offer medication counseling, medication therapy management, and medication review services to patients in underserved areas or remote locations. Telepharmacy allows patients to access clinical pharmacy services without physically visiting a pharmacy.
- Pharmacist-Managed Anticoagulation Clinic Model: Clinical pharmacists work in specialized anticoagulation clinics, monitoring and managing patients on anticoagulant therapy, such as warfarin or direct oral anticoagulants. They perform regular therapeutic monitoring, adjust dosages, provide patient education, and ensure appropriate follow-up to minimize complications and optimize therapy.
- Pediatric Clinical Pharmacy Model: Clinical pharmacists specializing in pediatric pharmacy provide specialized medication management and care for pediatric patients. They work collaboratively with pediatricians, pediatric nurses, and other healthcare professionals to optimize medication therapy, address specific pediatric medication needs, and ensure appropriate dosing and safety.
- Geriatric Clinical Pharmacy Model: Clinical pharmacists specializing in geriatric pharmacy focus on the unique medication needs and challenges faced by older adults. They provide comprehensive medication reviews, polypharmacy management, medication reconciliation, and medication education tailored to the specific needs of elderly patients.
- Oncology Pharmacy: Clinical pharmacists in oncology practice work as part of multidisciplinary oncology teams, providing specialized medication management for cancer patients. They assess chemotherapy regimens, manage supportive care medications, monitor for drug interactions and side effects, and provide patient education and counseling.

- ➤ Critical Care Pharmacy: Clinical pharmacists in critical care settings, such as intensive care units (ICUs), collaborate with healthcare teams to optimize medication therapy for critically ill patients. They provide dosing adjustments, manage complex medication regimens, monitor drug levels, and ensure medication safety in a high-acuity environment.
- ➤ Infectious Disease Pharmacy: Clinical pharmacists specializing in infectious diseases work closely with infectious disease physicians and healthcare teams to optimize antimicrobial therapy, prevent antibiotic resistance, and manage complex infectious disease cases. They provide expertise in dosing, monitoring, and antimicrobial stewardship.
- ➤ Mental Health Pharmacy: Clinical pharmacists in mental health settings collaborate with psychiatrists and mental health teams to optimize medication therapy for patients with mental health conditions. They assess medication regimens, monitor for side effects, provide medication education, and assist in treatment selection and adherence.
- ➤ Anticoagulation Clinic Pharmacy: Clinical pharmacists in anticoagulation clinics provide specialized care for patients on anticoagulant therapy, such as warfarin or direct oral anticoagulants. They monitor coagulation parameters, adjust doses, provide education on medication management, and ensure patient safety.
- ➤ These are just a few examples of clinical pharmacy practice models, and there are variations and combinations of these models depending on the practice setting and patient population. Clinical pharmacists can adapt and integrate different models to provide patient-centered and comprehensive medication management in various healthcare environments.

Appendix C: Survey Questionnaire for Clinical Pharmacists

Below is a sample survey questionnaire that can be used to gather information from clinical pharmacists. You can modify and customize it according to your specific research objectives and requirements.

1. Demographic Information:

   a. Age:

   b. Gender:

   c. Years of experience as a clinical pharmacist:

   d. Highest level of education:

   e. Current practice setting:

2. Clinical Pharmacy Practice:

   a. Describe your primary role and responsibilities as a clinical pharmacist.

   b. What specialized areas of clinical pharmacy do you practice in, if any?

   c. How do you collaborate with other healthcare professionals in your practice? Please provide examples.

   d. How do you communicate and coordinate care with other members of the healthcare team?

   e. Are there any challenges you face in your practice regarding collaboration and communication? If yes, please elaborate.

3. Technological Advancements in Clinical Pharmacy:

a. Which technological tools or systems do you use in your clinical pharmacy practice?

b. How have these technologies impacted your workflow, patient care, and medication management?

c. Have you encountered any challenges or barriers related to the implementation or use of technology in your practice? If yes, please explain.

4. Personalized Pharmacotherapy and Precision Medicine:

a. Are you involved in pharmacogenomics or personalized medicine initiatives in your practice?

b. How do you incorporate genetic information or biomarkers in medication therapy decisions?

c. What challenges, if any, have you faced in implementing personalized pharmacotherapy approaches?

5. Interprofessional Collaboration:

a. Describe your experience working as part of an interprofessional healthcare team.

b. What strategies do you employ to enhance collaboration and communication with other healthcare professionals?

c. What benefits or outcomes have you observed from effective interprofessional collaboration?

6. Emerging Roles and Opportunities:

a. Are you currently involved in any emerging roles within clinical pharmacy? If yes, please describe.

b. How do you see the field of clinical pharmacy evolving in the future? Are there any particular areas or roles you anticipate to be significant?

7. Contemporary Issues in Clinical Pharmacy:

a. What are the major contemporary issues or challenges you face in your clinical pharmacy practice?

b. Are there any specific areas related to medication safety, affordability, pharmaceutical industry influence, or patient adherence that you find particularly challenging?

c. Have you identified any strategies or initiatives to address these challenges?

8. Advocacy and Leadership:

a. Have you been involved in advocacy efforts to promote the role of clinical pharmacists or influence policy changes related to clinical pharmacy practice?

b. How do you demonstrate leadership within your practice or profession?

9. Professional Development and Training:

a. How do you stay updated with the latest developments and evidence-based practices in clinical pharmacy?

b. Have you pursued any additional education or training opportunities to enhance your clinical pharmacy skills and knowledge?

10. Suggestions for Improvement:

a. In your opinion, what areas or aspects of clinical pharmacy practice require further improvement or attention?

b. Do you have any suggestions for enhancing the integration of clinical pharmacists into healthcare teams or improving patient care outcomes?

Thank you for your participation in this survey. Your input is valuable for our research.

Emerging Trends in Clinical Pharmacy: Exploring the Evolving Landscape

www.ingramcontent.com/pod-product-compliance
Lightning Source LLC
Chambersburg PA
CBHW060856170526
45158CB00001B/375